Dealing with Diabetes Burnout

How to Recharge and Get Back on Track When You Feel Frustrated and Overwhelmed Living with Diabetes

Ginger Vieira

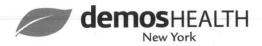

New York

Visit our website at www.demoshealth.com

ISBN: 978-1-936303-59-5
e-book ISBN: 978-1-61705-198-2

Acquisitions Editor: Julia Pastore
Compositor: diacriTech

Medical information provided by Demos Health, in the absence of a visit with a health care professional, must be considered as an educational service only. This book is not designed to replace a physician's independent judgment about the appropriateness or risks of a procedure or therapy for a given patient. Our purpose is to provide you with information that will help you make your own health care decisions.

The information and opinions provided here are believed to be accurate and sound, based on the best judgment available to the authors, editors, and publisher, but readers who fail to consult appropriate health authorities assume the risk of injuries. The publisher is not responsible for errors or omissions. The editors and publisher welcome any reader to report to the publisher any discrepancies or inaccuracies noticed.

Library of Congress Cataloging-in-Publication Data

Vieira, Ginger.
  Dealing with diabetes burnout : how to recharge and get back on track when you feel frustrated and overwhelmed living with diabetes / Ginger Vieira.
     pages cm
  Includes bibliographical references and index.
  ISBN 978-1-936303-59-5
1.   Diabetes—Popular works. I. Title. II. Title: Living with diabetes.
  RC660.4.V54 2014
  616.4'62—dc23
                                              2014000386

Special discounts on bulk quantities of Demos Health books are available to corporations, professional associations, pharmaceutical companies, health care organizations, and other qualifying groups. For details, please contact:

Special Sales Department
Demos Medical Publishing, LLC
11 West 42nd Street, 15th Floor
New York, NY 10036
Phone: 800-532-8663 or 212-683-0072
Fax: 212-941-7842
E-mail: specialsales@demosmedpub.com

Printed in the United States of America by McNaughton & Gunn.
14 15 16 17 18 / 5 4 3 2 1

Dealing with Diabetes Burnout

Also by Ginger Vieira
Emotional Eating with Diabetes
Your Diabetes Science Experiment

For Blue, Petey, and Einstein.
Thank you, my furry boys, for ensuring that each morning starts
with a walk in the woods and a smile.

"Diabetes doesn't define me, but it helps explain me."

—*Kerri Morrone Sparling, of SixUntilMe.com,*
living with type 1 diabetes

Contents

Acknowledgments

First, I can't help but thank my editor Julia Pastore for inviting me to create this book and giving me the utmost freedom to make it real, personal, and even silly and humorous.

I must also thank the Diabetes Online Community (DOC), for being this vast, vague, everywhere-and-anywhere community of people living with diabetes that is always nearby. When I asked you to share your experiences and stories, you shared. You are there for all of us during celebrations, disappointments, advocacy, sadness, humor, and much-needed venting. If anyone reading this book has yet to find the DOC, I urge you to type #DSMA into Twitter or join one of the dozens and dozens of Facebook groups for people with diabetes until you find a group or a few individuals who you connect with. Just say "Hello! I'm looking to meet other people with diabetes," and you'll find yourself surrounded online with support and new friends. We are not alone. Thank you to the hundreds—make that *thousands*—of individuals who live with their diabetes out loud, across the globe, in a community where we can all reach other.

Lastly, thank you to Roger and Tara, the two greatest sources of support that a girl could ask for in life with diabetes. Without either of you, this would be so much harder.

Love and gratitude,

Ginger

Introduction

The Perfect Diabetic ... I'd Rather Search for Bigfoot!

Have you ever wanted to be one of those *perfect diabetics*? Me, too. As people living with diabetes, we can't help but compare ourselves to that "perfect patient" our doctors, parents, boyfriends, wives, strangers, and friends all want us to become. There is an unspoken expectation to be flawless in all things despite the fact that such perfection is impossible.

Since the day I was diagnosed with type 1 diabetes in 1999, I have never met one of those elusive diabetics who gets it right all the time. I've met people with diabetes who work *really hard* to have the tightest blood sugar control possible, but even they haven't attained perfection. Even they have moments or days when their blood sugars are higher or lower than perfect, when they eat something that a "diabetic shouldn't eat," when they forget to check their blood sugar before a meal, when they can't find time to exercise, or when they miscount the total carbohydrates in their grandmother's all-natural, whole grain, homemade bread and thus, take too much insulin.

I've also met people with diabetes who try really hard to do the best they can do, and people with diabetes who are sincerely struggling to find the motivation to take care of themselves, and perfection seems as illusive and mysterious as Big Foot. Or unicorns. (My sincerest apologies go out to those who are still waiting for a unicorn sighting.)

And that's okay, because this disease—type 1, type 2, and type 1.5—is really hard work.

From the moment we are diagnosed with *any* type of diabetes, we begin a part of our lives in which we are constantly graded. Constantly tested. Constantly told whether we're doing a great job, a good job, an okay job, or a *really bad* job based on the numbers that show up on our glucose meter and A1C test. We are graded on what we eat or on how often we exercise.

Whether we check our blood sugar regularly or rarely, and somewhere in our heads we can't help but tell ourselves that we're "good" or "bad" based entirely on how well we are able to accomplish this neverending to-do list throughout every single day.

And that is exhausting.

It can go something like this: I'm "good" for checking my blood sugar at least four times a day, but I'm "bad" for going too many hours, or even days, without checking. I'm "good" for drinking water. I'm "bad" for drinking a martini. I'm "good" for eating steamed chicken and vegetables. I'm "bad" for eating ice cream and cookies. I'm "good" for being able to accurately count the carbohydrates in my dinner, and dose my insulin for that meal, but I'm "bad" if my estimated carb-count is off by even 5 or 10 grams and my blood sugar is high as a result.

And I'm definitely a *bad, bad, bad* diabetic if I eat a chocolate peanut butter cup. (I love peanut butter cups, and any candy that is fruity, sour, and is dyed the color red. Does my sweet-tooth make me a "bad" diabetic?) But hey, I also *really* love asparagus, chicken, strawberries, and almond butter, but high-fives for making good decisions don't seem to be nearly as forthcoming as raised eyebrows and gasps for "bad decisions."

Everything we do or don't do, choose or don't choose, inevitably leads to criticism of how well we are taking care of our diabetes. Sometimes the criticism comes directly from our own heads, and sometimes it comes from our doctor or the people who love us.

If you've ever been diagnosed with a complication of diabetes, you've inevitably wondered, "Did I do this to myself?" Blaming yourself can lead to feelings of guilt and even self-punishment. And if you've ever had an A1C test come back higher than you hoped for, even if your health care team is supportive, you've probably felt a sense of failure, "Well, I didn't do it right this time! Once again, fail!"

But we *don't* need to do it perfectly in order to be doing an amazing job in life with diabetes. Seriously.

I bet if you actually read the very long "diabetes to-do list" aloud to your health care team, your mother, your boyfriend, or best friend, they would probably say, "Well, yeah, I don't expect you to do all of those things perfectly! *That's crazy!* I can't even do those things perfectly as a *non*-diabetic!"

And then you might even read all of that aloud to yourself, and very logically think, "Well, yeah, I shouldn't expect myself to be perfect in all of those things! I deserve the freedom to make mistakes! *Geez Louise! Good grief! Holy moly! Gadzooks!"*

Even though we may intellectually know that these expectations are unrealistic, we still blame ourselves for our mistakes and shortcomings over and over and over. We still feel that constant, unspoken pressure to be flawless. This pressure sits on all our shoulders—all day long—and it can effortlessly transform itself into guilt, blame, self-sabotage, and hopelessness. Wrap all of those things together and you're left feeling *totally burned-out.*

Totally ready to give up.

But you can officially know for sure that you are *not* the only person experiencing this burnout! Trust me, there are many others who are feeling some version of what you're feeling.

I'm writing this book because I want you to know that you are not alone and that you don't have to be perfect. I want to help you put an end to the guilt-tripping, blaming, and scolding, and instead learn how to set yourself up for success, and feel proud of yourself for facing diabetes every day even when the numbers on your meter aren't as perfect as you'd like them be.

This book is about putting into words what all of you may feel now, a few years from now, or may have felt in the past ever since your diagnosis. We're going to look at why burnout happens, how to be okay with it, and how to move through it, eventually finding yourself back on your feet. But there's more to living well with diabetes than just the emotional aspects, right? And part of lessening our burnout is about feeling more prepared to take on the actual tasks of managing diabetes every day. And *believing* in our abilities to face diabetes every day.

We're going to talk about how to make real progress in the three things that impact diabetes most: blood sugar management, nutrition, and exercise. I'll provide real tips and suggestions for real changes. With compassion, knowledge, and humor, this book will provide you with the tools and support you need to feel empowered and encouraged to never give up.

I've lived with type 1 diabetes and celiac disease since 1999, and I would give it back in a heartbeat. I would sell both these diseases at a yard sale in trade for *nothing* or maybe for the going price for an old VHS tape, which last I checked costs about 35 cents. And yes, one day they may find a cure—and that will be an awesome day—but until that day, my goal is to not only live healthfully but also *happily*. To thrive, not just to survive. Diabetes may get to use up a tremendous amount of my mental energy every day, but I refuse to let it use up my happiness!

On a daily basis, I am trying to balance three things: diabetes, life, and happiness. Life doesn't stop just because my blood sugar is suddenly low. And my blood sugar doesn't care that while it's inconveniently low I'm actually trying to workout in the gym or speak at a conference or enjoy a movie with my fella or hike in the woods with my dogs. Diabetes does not care.

And then there's the happiness part.

Is attaining that magical state of "diabetic perfection" worth it if my entire existence revolves around trying to have perfect—and I mean *perfect*—blood sugars … even if it comes with endless stress and overwhelming pressure? I don't think so. Part of the balancing act is about learning how to "roll with the punches" of diabetes, like forgiving myself quickly for the high blood sugar I had yesterday morning because I treated a severe low blood sugar in the middle of the night with two juice boxes, 30 grams of carbohydrates, instead of just 15. Correct, learn the lesson—a 35 mg/dL in the middle of the night does *not* actually need two juice boxes despite how scarily sweaty and shaky I was at the time—and move on.

The balancing act is also about knowing when it's time to ease up on diabetes management for the sake of enjoying something in life that wouldn't be nearly as fun if I was overly concerned about having perfect blood sugars. You really think I'm *never* going to eat cotton candy again at the state fair just because it's not "ideal" for people with diabetes? No, that's not necessary. It's a treat—and we'll talk about this later—but you can bet your bottom dollar I still make room in my life for things like cotton candy.

Now believe me, I have days, weeks, and sometimes just overwhelming moments when diabetes makes me mad, frustrated, and sad, but those phases of burnout don't stop me from living the life I want to live. And I want to show you how to create that balance for yourself. To feel burned-out and not only be okay with it, but move *through it* at your very own pace.

Okay? Okay. Let's do it. You are not in this alone!

Dealing with Diabetes Burnout

No Vacations or Days Off? This Is the Worst Job Ever!

Exploring the Pressures and Expectations That Can Make Diabetes Feel So Darn Overwhelming

So this is the part of the book where I try to convince you that living with diabetes *can* be fun and easy! *Cough. Cough.* *I'm just kidding*. Seriously. In reality, there are sort of positive consequences that come from this diagnosis, but I wouldn't really go as far to call them "benefits." Sure, many people find diabetes to be an awesome inspiration for learning more about food and exercise, or an incredible way to meet new people through the greater diabetes online community, but would most of us trade those "benefits" in a heartbeat if it meant we could simply *not* have diabetes? You betcha!

Living with diabetes isn't fun. It's hard work, except even the word "work" doesn't really cover it. Diabetes makes any normal "work" look like a totally awesome party.

Imagine for a moment that your best friend is telling you about her new "job": she's required to show up to work every single day of the week. Monday through Sunday, even on Christmas and her birthday. Her workday starts the moment she wakes up every morning, and not a minute later. (And no, she can't call in to say she'll be late because of a snowstorm or a flat tire—her new job doesn't care.)

Instead of a lunch break, she's expected to work even harder during meals, even snacks. If she uses her lunch break to go to a yoga class or for a bike ride, she has to actually work harder. Holidays, like Thanksgiving Day, and parties are a nightmare—not a moment of celebration can go by without having to think about her job.

She's also been warned that her new job can be very dangerous. Even when she's doing her best, this job can land her in the hospital, cause seizures or comas, cause really bad sick days, and eventually, someday, her eyesight, the health of her fingers and toes, and some of her organs might even be in jeopardy. But even throughout all of *that* or after she's home from the hospital, she doesn't get a break from her job.

And when does her workday end? Never, really. She comes home from her day job and keeps working at home. She gets ready for bed, and keeps working. And while she's sleeping, at least some part of her mind needs to keep working to make sure everything goes smoothly.

None of that sounds like any "work" I've done over the years while being employed at movie theaters, gyms, restaurants, advertising agencies, yada yada yada. Not a single one of those places made me work all day, every day, even when I was sick with the flu!

With a "job" like that, would you blame your friend for having occasional days where she just can't keep up with all of her responsibilities? The pressure? Would you blame her for getting totally and completely frustrated? So frustrated that she wants to quit her job as soon as possible, or at least not show up for a few days, even if it means putting her life in danger?

Living with diabetes is *crazy hard work*—every single day—and there are no breaks, no vacations, no days off. There isn't even an hour off here or there. Even when we're doing a great job and our blood sugar is a shining example of great diabetes management, we're working *intensely* to make it happen. The smoothest blood sugar levels are not the result of something that has become "easy" to manage, but instead, they are the result of dedication, commitment, sweat, and maybe even tears!

(And sometimes those "perfect days" are even a fluke that we can't explain, which can be annoyingly wonderful. Even more irritating are the days when we're doing everything right and our numbers imply that we're doing everything *so* wrong! Roar! But we'll talk about that later.)

How often do you simply *think* about your blood sugar? The moment you wake up? After breakfast? While you're walking from the subway to your office building? While you're clothes shopping with your children? While you're making out with your girlfriend or trying to celebrate the New Year at your best friend's party?

It's endless. Whether or not you become noticeably frustrated with your diabetes, the constant thought, energy, and worry is inevitable. And *that* can lead to burnout. That constant effort and worry is exhausting, even if it motivates you to take care of yourself.

Despite the demands of diabetes and the immense list of responsibilities that even many doctors probably couldn't keep up with themselves, we still *scold* ourselves for getting overwhelmed, for getting tired, for *not* being the perfect diabetic machine.

When you think about everything that living with diabetes entails, and the nonstop expectations and responsibilities, I would actually be more surprised if you *didn't* get burned-out, frustrated, and tired of managing diabetes. In fact, we should actually *anticipate and expect* that every now and then, whether it's every few years or every few months, we will experience at least *a little* burnout.

So, what *is* diabetes burnout?

Diabetes Burnout Can Be Round, Purple, Tall, or Covered in Spots

It's hard to give just one definition for "diabetes burnout" because what that looks like in your life compared to mine or anyone else's can be drastically different. And the phase of burnout you feel this year could be very different from a phase of burnout you experience seven years from now. This year it could be about occasionally skipping your insulin doses, while seven years from now it could be about just feeling really down and stressed even though you're doing everything a "perfect diabetic" would do. There is no specific behavior, length of time, or intensity of burnout that qualifies it as "real burnout." Your own experience is your own burnout, and later in the chapter, you'll describe what burnout looks like in your life.

First, let's try to give some clarity to what "diabetes burnout" *can or might* look like. Keep in mind that the following examples can qualify as "burnout" whether they last for a day, a week, or a dozen years:

- Feeling sick and tired of diabetes management as a whole because it's never-ending
- Lying to your parents about your blood sugars because they won't wanna hear the real digits
- Eating lots and lots of candy (or some carbohydrate-packed food) just to spite your diabetes
- Drinking lots and lots of soda, beer, and cocktails because everybody's always telling you not to drink those things
- Feeling like you want to give up completely
- Going a few days without taking your oral meds, or taking them hours later than scheduled
- Purposely running your blood sugars high because the idea of experiencing another low blood sugar is too stressful, scary, and really inconvenient
- Being careless with carbohydrate-counting because you just don't have the energy to measure it all out and do the required math for insulin dosing every day
- Avoiding fresh vegetables and fruits because you know they're good for you but you're so tired of everybody telling you to be a "good diabetic"
- Feeling stressed-out and frustrated because you can't figure out why your blood sugar is always high after dinner (or lunch or breakfast or whenever!)
- Feeling annoyed that you're the only person in your classroom/office/ house who has to poke their fingers, take injections, take pills, and watch every little gram of what they eat all day long
- Spending a week wallowing in sadness after being told by the eye doctor that your retinopathy has progressed or being diagnosed with neuropathy or any other complication
- Feeling frustrated with trying to manage something that doesn't have a perfect solution, always presents new variables, and constantly disrupts your day
- Hardly ever checking your blood sugar, if at all, because you just don't freakin' want to

- Taking just enough insulin to barely keep yourself alive
- Feeling constantly angry and drained around the everyday work you do to live a healthy life with diabetes

To feel burned-out in diabetes management doesn't necessarily mean that you're not taking care of yourself. Instead, it can simply mean that while you go about checking your blood sugar, counting your carbs, taking your oral meds, and taking your insulin, you feel incredibly stressed-out and tired. For others, diabetes burnout can absolutely mean you're neglecting your blood sugars, harming your body, and struggling so much on an emotional level that you're putting your physical health in danger. And then there's somewhere in between: where your body isn't exactly in grave danger because of your burnout, but you're definitely not making diabetes a priority, and your blood sugars are paying the price.

All forms of burnout matter because how you feel matters, and most importantly, *you* matter.

Let's take a look at what others have to say about diabetes burnout in their lives. The following statements have been shared with me through an anonymous survey, from people of all ages with type 1 and type 2 diabetes:

When I feel burned-out on diabetes...

"I skip it all—pricks, boluses. I seem to block it out and forget. Then I work hard at it again and try, then skip and forget, and repeat."

∽

"I just want to unplug from my pump, eat what I want, and have the freedom of not wondering 'Am I okay?' all the time."

∽

"I don't check my blood sugar. I completely ignore my meter and my pump and just pretend. Until I feel so sick that I have to act. I've been doing this for 14 years, on and off."

(continued)

(continued)

When I feel burned-out on diabetes...

"I will basically go on 'Diabetes Vacation.' I stop giving myself insulin and checking my blood sugars. I get really lazy and don't care. When it happens, it's on the weekend or during breaks off from school. After a few days of skipping most of my insulin and feeling sick, I realize that I'm only hurting myself and get back on track."

∞

"I don't want to do another injection, another finger-prick, see the doctor again, fight to pick up my prescription, look at carbohydrate counts, exercise, think about or do anything related to diabetes because everything changes my sugars. I just don't want to have to deal with any of it anymore. Mentally or physically. I just want to go to bed and sleep all day long and never get up and have to deal with it. But then I have to because otherwise my sugars spike and I feel lousy."

∞

"I get discouraged after a high number, and I find it really gets me down trying to figure out where I went wrong or what I did to deserve it."

∞

"I feel completely overwhelmed that this is for life."

∞

"I eat. Candy."

∞

"Early on, around year four of diabetes, I actually went on an insulin strike—no shots, no testing, no nothing! That didn't last long! More recently, I'll binge on carbs and take a sh*tload of insulin to cover."

(continued)

(continued)

When I feel burned-out on diabetes...

"I haven't seen an endocrinologist in about eight years. I am fed up with seeing doctors all the time and being made to feel as though it was 'my fault' for not having perfect blood sugars. I am so over diabetes, so sick of the lows and highs. I still try and manage it by testing and eating right, and I see a general physician for insulin prescriptions, but I don't micromanage it in the way I used to. After 30 years, I'm fed up with it and accept I'll have a reduced life expectancy. I've made my peace with that."

∞

"I feel resentful about counting carbs ... and skipping boluses or doses because I just didn't want to deal with it."

∞

"I eat really sugary foods and don't bolus properly for them."

∞

"When I am burned-out, I don't test, just guess again on the carb-count and hope for the best. This doesn't last too long because I feel tired and then test and correct. Lots of times when people are bugging me, I wish they had it so they would see it's not as simple as taking medicine!"

∞

"When I'm burned out I eat whatever I want!"

∞

"I feel frustrated when I do everything right and I still have high blood sugar. I feel resentful that I have to pay so much money for supplies that I rely on to live and to stay healthy. I feel resentful and fed up when I have to hurt myself when replacing my pump inset, especially when I have to do it twice in one day due to not finding a good site.

(continued)

(continued)

When I feel burned-out on diabetes...

"I'm resentful that I have scars all over my thighs and hips because of my pump."

∾

"Not bolusing, not checking, eventually going into DKA [diabetic ketoacidosis]."

∾

"I 'quit' being diabetic as a teenager. I ate what I wanted, refused injections for days at a time, causing severe DKA multiple times a year. My attitude and habits have since changed, but I still get angry about having to do the little things like finger pricks and set changes for my pump when I'm tired."

∾

"I felt burned-out after I spent two years losing weight and really watching my diabetes. Then all of my friends told me I was spending too much time thinking about what I eat and that I was addicted to food because of it. That mixed message didn't help either because I was already so tired of dealing with my health. There was that daily routine with diabetes, but also with my other illnesses as well. I had 18 other medications to take in addition to asthma, migraines, depression, chronic back disease, and blood pressure problems to contend with. One day, I just didn't take any of my medications. I became so tired and upset that I stopped caring what I ate and soon gained back the weight I had lost. Now, I realize it might have been burnout as well as anger at myself and others."

∾

"When I am burned-out after five failed insulin pump sites, I may throw my pump (onto a soft surface; you don't need a broken pump as well) and ignore it until my blood sugar gets too high."

(continued)

(continued)

When I feel burned-out on diabetes...

"For me, I slack off and don't test at all."

∞

"I stop checking for a day or two. If I'm sick of dealing with low after low (especially at night) I'll purposefully run my numbers higher."

∞

"Diabetes burnout for me is not wanting to prick my fingers. Not wanting to count carbs. Not wanting to insert numbers into my insulin pump. Diabetes burnout is not wanting to eat because of the millions of little things you have to do before taking a bite. My diabetes burnout goes hand in hand with diabetes depression. I want to just curl up in bed and not do a single thing. But in the end I have to do it anyway. Even if I decide to do nothing, if I decide to take a break from the busyness of the world ... I still need to prick my finger and face the number that comes up on that little screen. Because I know that even if I don't do anything physically, my numbers can still get out of control. So sometimes, even though I don't want to deal with a single aspect of diabetes, I take a deep breath and let a few tears roll down my cheeks, then I just carry on with the realities of my life."

∞

"I get tired of all of it. Often. I plow through because I know I must. Since I've had type 1 diabetes for over 45 years, I learned far different care and eating methods at diagnosis than are practiced today. Then I used shots, now called MDI's, but often it was ODI— one daily injection vs. multiple. Now I use the pump after many years of trying to determine to go on it. I tested my urine with a test tube. I counted calories and exchanges. Now, of course, because so much has been studied and learned, it is multiple daily blood sticks and counting carbs. It is the 365/24/7 (366 during leap years) that is the drudgery.

(continued)

(continued)

When I feel burned-out on diabetes...

"Burnout means not testing like I should, not bolusing like I should, not counting carbs like I should ... all the time. That is burnout. Is there never a moment at this stage that I do not feel burnout? I do not think so."

ॐ

"Tired of always having to count carbs before I can eat! Always thinking about food!! What I can and can't have!"

ॐ

"I still take my blood sugar all the time and give myself insulin. I just binge on sweets."

ॐ

"For me, diabetic burnout has included tears, angry poetry, resentfulness. I've often not checked my blood sugars regularly or gone without bolusing correctly ... or sometimes at all!"

ॐ

"I feel as though no matter how hard I try, it's impossible to achieve well-rounded numbers."

ॐ

"I get upset when I find out there is yet another medical problem associated with diabetes, and some of them I can develop no matter how well I take care of myself."

ॐ

"There are so many treats that seem even more appealing to me now than they ever did before. I want to be able to eat whatever I want, but I remain strict with my diet."

(continued)

(*continued*)

When I feel burned-out on diabetes...

"*Angry. Angry at everything, especially those that take their (or seem to) health for granted!*"

∽

"*I accept that my life span will be a little shorter than other healthy people.*"

∽

"*I drink.*"

∽

"*I feel extremely guilty all the time. I also blame diabetes for everything that is wrong in my life.*"

∽

"*Sometimes I wake up and I say to myself 'Why am I the one who has to have this?'*"

∽

"*The fact that it never goes away, and you can't forget about it.*"

The Tips of My Fingers Really %*$*# Hurt!

Literally, as I type this, a bit of blood just appeared on my computer keyboard from the last time I checked my blood sugar, hardly 20 minutes ago. And that reminds me of the one part of diabetes management that personally annoys me the most: the constant pricking of my fingers.

This is what *my* burnout looks like. At least, it's how my burnout has taken shape this year. It's not huge, not devastating ... but it's a daily occurrence, a daily thought, that has been weighing on my shoulders recently.

Advertisements for glucose meters and "painless lancet devices" always make me angry. They all hurt, eventually. When you have a bajillion holes in your fingers, it doesn't matter how amazingly brilliant your lancet device is—it's going to hurt when it's stabbing fingers covered in old wounds.

Like yours, my 10 fingers have been through a lot. (Well, actually, I don't use my thumbs—I don't know why—so it's only eight fingers that endure the abuse.) The 15 years of type 1 diabetes I've experienced so far has led to an average of six finger pricks each day. That's almost 33,000 total sharp objects stabbing the tips of my fingers, all for the sake of my health in life with diabetes. (And that doesn't even include the insulin injections, which adds up to at least 27,375 more sharp object stabbings so far, if you were wondering!)

Individually, all of those finger pricks are no big deal, right? They're tiny, and they hurt for merely a moment, if at all. But those eight fingers are *covered* in little black spots—scabs, really—from those 33,000 finger pricks, and sometimes they *really*, genuinely hurt. Sometimes the tips of my fingers get so sore and sensitive, and the idea of stabbing my finger again just makes me kind of angry. Sometimes I have to prick two or three fingers just to find an area that isn't so calloused that it will finally bleed. I can only imagine what it's like for little kids, whose fingertips are half the size of mine.

(And sure, there are continuous glucose monitors (CGMs)—I wear one now—but it's not like CGMs are placed with the kisses from kittens and heart-shaped stickers. Those, too, involve puncturing your flesh, and can leave plenty of beat-up tissue with scars and bruising. And wearing a CGM doesn't mean you don't have to also prick your finger!)

Of course, there are so many things much worse in the world than enduring more finger pricks, I know. But for me, that is one part of diabetes management that is an ongoing thing that irks me—sometimes in a big way, sometimes just a little.

Does it keep me from pricking my fingers?

Well, no, because my desire to know my blood sugar is much greater than my annoyance with all the little spots on my fingertips. I've taught myself to have this conversation, whenever I need to overcome that annoyance with pricking my fingers:

> **Burned-out Ginger:** *I'm so sick of pricking my finger. It hurts sometimes, and it's so annoying.*
>
> **Other Ginger:** *But I need to know what my blood sugar is.*
>
> **Burned-out Ginger:** *Why? What does it matter right now? It's just gonna be another damn hole in one of your eight overly poked fingers. Bleh. No, thanks.*
>
> **Other Ginger:** *Listen, I know it's hard, and it sometimes really sucks to deal with this every day, and that's okay. I don't blame you for being tired of it.*
>
> **Burned-out Ginger:** *Good, then don't do it. Don't deal with diabetes today. Diabetes sucks.*
>
> **Other Ginger:** *But if I don't do it, I won't know what my blood sugar is right now. I won't know if I need more insulin, some glucose, or nothing at all. I need to know that so the day goes as smoothly as possible, so my A1C is as close to my goal as possible, so I can respond to the number and take care of myself, because I want to feel good!*
>
> **Burned-out Ginger:** *Ugh! Fine. Whatever. Just go ahead and get it over with.*

Creating that conversation, making it a habit in my head, and getting from the beginning of that conversation to the end of that conversation took time to develop. And that's all it is really: a habit that I've created in how I think about my diabetes when I'm feeling less than inspired to deal with all the tedious responsibilities that come with it. And we'll talk about this more when developing your Mental Skills Toolbox in Chapter 2.

But first, we have to express what we're feeling. Right now. Today.

What is the source of *your burnout*, and what does *your burnout* feel like?

If you need a little help digging into those details, give the following exercise a try:

Pretend You're Being Interviewed by Barbara Walters (or Jimmy Fallon or Chelsea Handler or Oprah or Charlie Rose or Elmo!)

If you're anything like me, you probably don't feel like telling your boyfriend or your mom about how much you hate diabetes. I mean, sure, we can express to those who love us how we feel sometimes, but they will never really understand how it feels if they don't also live with diabetes. Venting to my mom will just make her feel upset that her youngest child has to live with this chronic illness every day, and my fiance, Roger, hasn't had to go to a doctor in about 17 years, so it's hard for him to relate.

Talking about your diabetes *to* someone might not be as important as simply talking about it *out loud* to nobody. In other words, the next time you're on a long drive or alone at home, pretend you're being interviewed by Barbara Walters and **let it all out.**

The value of expressing how you really feel is an incredibly important part of working through your burnout. Being able to genuinely *feel* what you *feel*, instead of feeling as if you need to hide it from the world, can be the most significant step you take in moving forward.

If I were being interviewed by Barbara Walters, in my imagination, here's how I imagine it might go:

> **Barb:** *So, Ginger, what makes you feel the most angry about diabetes?*
>
> **Ginger:** *Honestly, Barb, I really $%*&$%* hate having to wear diabetes technology, and I don't even wear any today! But the idea of it makes me angry. I wore a pump for the first seven years of my*

life with diabetes, and then I suddenly just started hating it. I've been taking shots for the past eight years. The idea that "optimal blood glucose control" is only attainable by wearing something in my skin all day … just makes me furious.

Barb: *But pump technology is supposed to make life with diabetes better, right?*

Ginger: *Sure, and for a lot of people it does, but not for me. I tried going back on the pump briefly once, and I test-drove a continuous glucose monitor, and I was just suddenly furious. The feeling of it in my skin, ugh, it made me so angry. I hate that the highest level of technology today still involves jamming a skinny cannula into my flesh and wearing it every single day. It leaves holes and scars, and sometimes those scars get itchy and irritated. And there's blood that kinks the tubing, which causes high blood sugars and ketones and … geez. Pumps are great, sure, but they aren't perfect, and personally, they just make me angry. And ya know what, my blood sugars are great without all that technology!*

Barb: *Okay, I hear you. What else makes you angry about diabetes?*

Ginger: *Oh, Barb, honey, I don't know how much time you've got, but have I mentioned how much my fingers seem to hurt on a daily basis these days? I mean, like, every time I check my blood sugar, I hesitate! I actually hesitate after 15 years of diabetes and an average of six finger-pricks a day because it's starting to hurt so much. How will my fingers feel in another 15 years? I can't imagine.*

Barb: *Oh dear, I'm sorry to hear that, Ginger. Keep going.*

Ginger: *Well …*

I think you get the point, right? Barbara Walters and I are talking about my *feelings*, my *worries*, my *stress* around my life with diabetes. Sure, having a real-life human to listen and respond can be wonderful, too, but you might not have that kind of person in your life. Simply talking out loud and giving your feelings a chance to be expressed is important. So whether you're being interviewed by Barbara Walters, Jon Stewart, Oprah Winfrey, or Regis Philbin, **let yourself express and _feel_ what you truly actually feel!**

If you need somewhere to get started with a pencil and paper, go for it:

_____

_____

_____

_____

_____

_____

_____

_____

Learning to Express the Little Things!

Sometimes, it's just the little things that build up on a daily basis that can feel the most overwhelming, especially if you don't know anyone else living with diabetes who "gets it." Instead, finding someone who will listen to how frustrated and overwhelmed you are in any given moment, who you can easily text or call or e-mail three sentences to, can be priceless.

Somebody who will listen without judgment, without telling you something like, "Well, at least it's not cancer" or something equally irritating or dismissive. Tell somebody who will listen and then say something like, "I don't blame you, living with diabetes seems like it might be really hard some days."

For example, the other afternoon around 4:00 p.m. I had a low blood sugar of 45 mg/dL. I had spent most of the day outside gardening and pulling weeds, which I planned for by consuming some juice throughout the afternoon to prevent any lows, but several hours after I'd relaxed in front of a movie, the hours of gardening caught up with blood sugar and I was low. Bleh—oh well.

So I treated my low with grapes. I didn't count them out, but I also didn't go hog wild and eat the whole bowl. I ate what seemed like a very reasonable amount of grapes in order to treat my low, approximately 15 to 25 grams of carbs. Two hours later, moments before I should have started preparing dinner for my family, I realized I felt really thirsty, sort of nauseated, and not at all hungry, considering it had been several hours since I'd eaten a real meal.

To make a long story short: those grapes caused my blood sugar to spike to 350 mg/dL.

"Ughh!" I groaned.

"What's wrong?" asked Roger as he looked over my shoulder at my meter.

"I don't want diabetes anymore. I'm so sick of it."

He didn't need to speak in order to support me. Instead, he gave me a kiss, and the look in his eyes told me, "I totally hate that you have to deal with this disease every day and I wish I could make it go away." (What he *didn't* do, thankfully, was gasp at the number on my meter or scold me for somehow eating too many grapes, but we'll talk more about that stuff in Chapter 7.)

And then the moment passed … well, sort of. Sure, I continued to be incredibly irritated while cooking dinner because high blood sugars leave me with zero appetite, and I knew I *hadn't* actually eaten an absurd amount of grapes so the high blood sugar just seemed unfair. But I didn't hold it in. I didn't hide it from Roger or put on a happy face. I expressed how frustrated I was in that moment to someone who could hear it. (Teaching those close to you "how to hear it" is a special process that we'll talk about in Chapter 7, I promise.)

Was that moment of diabetes a big deal that I couldn't take care? No, not at all, it was just another high blood sugar that I knew how to correct with an insulin dose, but it's the daily weight of dealing with diabetes that can wear on us. Sometimes that weight looks like an emergency, and sometimes it's so subtle on the outside that the people around us don't even know we're under that weight.

But that daily weight of *thinking* about your blood sugars, *thinking* about what we're eating, and *thinking* about exercise is subtle but exhausting. You can't tell by looking at me that I spend probably 60 percent of my mental energy on thinking about my blood sugar, trying to make good choices around food, making sure my blood sugar behaves when I exercise, and remembering to take the right amount of insulin at the right times of day.

That subtle stress needs to come out. Somehow. Somewhere. To someone. An anonymous pen pal, a real-life friend you can meet on a Saturday afternoon, or a paid mental health professional—any of the above might well make the cut. With the day-to-day tedious weight of diabetes, talking about it all can feel like a release. You let it go. It gets out. You no longer have to carry it in your mind—at least for a little while. Maybe down the road, you might find you need to unload some of that weight again.

Moving Forward

In the next chapter, we're going to look below the surface of our emotions around diabetes burnout and look at the specific behavior and actions of our burnout, and how those actions can impact our entire life, not just our diabetes.

I Haven't Checked My Blood Sugar in Three Weeks (ehh … Months)

2

Digging Deeper into What Is Currently Happening in Your Life with Diabetes

So you want to *overcome* your burnout, right? I'm sure you'd like to skip right ahead to that part of your life where the sun is shining and you're full of inspired motivation to be an "almost-perfect" diabetic, but there's a little bit of digging we need to do first. (Actually, it'd be nice if we could all skip ahead to the day "they" find a cure, but let's not get too carried away!)

Before you try to "get over" something, it's important to really understand where you're starting from and what's currently going on in your life (and your head) around your diabetes. Just like planning a cross-country road trip, you can't start driving to get there until you know the location where you're starting from (and, of course, where you *really* want to go). Digging deeper into your burnout is about being very honest with how you are currently managing your diabetes on a day-to-day basis, how you're eating, how you're taking your insulin and exercising. Digging deeper is about creating a very clear understanding of what life with diabetes looks like in your actions and behaviors today *before* trying to move forward and achieve a specific goal.

There are two key things I'd like you to keep in mind while you read this chapter and begin to acknowledge the details of your diabetes burnout:

1. You *should not* feel as though you must overcome your burnout today, tomorrow, or even next month. It's a process, and that process can take a short amount of time or a longer amount of time—and that's okay. Your experience is your own.

2. Overcoming burnout this month or this year does not mean you or anyone else should expect that you will never encounter burnout again in the future. You're human, and until they find a cure to help this ol' pancreas, you have every right to experience burnout.

We talked in Chapter 1 about the many forms of burnout, but this chapter is about *your burnout.* The nitty-gritty details that make your thoughts and your feelings about diabetes all your own. Acknowledging the true details of your burnout is critical. Writing those details down—and maybe even sharing them with someone—brings those feelings into reality. Most importantly, though, truly acknowledging what is fueling your burnout is going to help you create a new way of thinking about or managing that part of your life with diabetes.

Let's start with the *small* moments of burnout first.

It's Just a Bad Day for Diabetes

Sometimes, burnout might feel like too big of a word for what you're feeling. Or maybe you feel like you get momentary thoughts of burnout that last for 12 seconds until you're distracted by your dog or your daughter or a text message. Sometimes there are days, Bad Days for Diabetes, when that number on your glucose meter seems to be laughing at you, cackling even, because everything you do in an effort to get your blood sugar back on track just doesn't seem to be working. It feels like, for 24 hours, you just can't win. And it feels like the day will never end.

The world we live in doesn't exactly support life with diabetes. There's junk food around every corner. If you have kids or a hectic job, there isn't a worldwide freebie for people with diabetes so we can ensure we eat our meals on time or have a spare moment to check our blood sugar or take our meds. Less healthy food is cheaper. Having time for exercise certainly isn't a big priority on your boss's mind. And the chaos of life really doesn't care if it leaves you with the mental energy to remember to check your blood sugar. Oh, and not every food in the world comes with a nutrition panel in order to count carbohydrates—the healthiest foods often don't come in packages at all!

But the biggest issue of all is that we're being asked to manage something our body is supposed to do all on its own based on a variety of other physiological and hormonal and yada yada yada processes! And we *cannot* do it perfectly. Which means some days just get thrown way off course and it can take the entire rest of the day to catch up.

And *that* is a bad day for diabetes. You just feel stuck there, waiting until the horrible ride ends and you can get back to your "norm." Whether it's a series of high blood sugars, a bad batch of insulin, rebounding from a really bad low blood sugar, or maybe you were trying to enjoy a day with your family and the frosting on that cupcake was a real whammy, or perhaps you just feel like no matter what you do, you're three steps behind and you won't catch up until the next day.

That's a bad day with diabetes. And it happens to all of us! It's exhausting, draining, frustrating, guilt-tripping, and it's a reality we face because we *can't* do it all perfectly. And we definitely can't structure every aspect of our lives to be totally perfect for diabetes because that's just a totally crazy expectation! The world, unfortunately, doesn't revolve around our blood sugar needs! Oh my, how nice that would be.

A few moments of diabetes that can make the day feel neverending or just *really* annoying:

- When you've changed the infusion set for your insulin pump three times and the insulin still isn't getting through
- Pricking your finger over and over and over and over
- When you just desperately want to fall asleep on the couch until you remember you need to check your blood sugar and take your long-acting insulin dose or pills
- When your insulin expires and leads to high blood sugars that you think are your fault until the end of the day, when you realize the insulin expired
- Heading to the gym only to realize your blood sugar is low by the time you get there … which completely ruins your workout plans!
- When you just want to enjoy a cup of popcorn at the movies with your friends, but you have to use the light from your phone to find your insulin pen and take the right amount of insulin in the dark theater

- When you're on a first date and your blood sugar is through the roof, and you feel nauseous, but you're still trying to put on a happy face for your date!
- When your flight home is delayed, you've run out of oral meds, you need to spend the night in the airport, you miss your next dose, and you're guaranteed to have a very high blood sugar by morning
- When you're on vacation eating food you've never eaten before, attempting to guess impossible-to-guess carbohydrate counts, and trying to enjoy your vacation while your blood sugar goes up and down like it's jumping on a pogo stick
- When you're in Italy and you accidentally spill all of your test-strips into a puddle while you're two hours from your hotel on a day-long winery tour
- When you eat a really big buffet breakfast with your family on Christmas morning only to spend the rest of the day battling high blood sugars
- When your blood sugar seems to be stuck at 45 mg/dL and you cannot get it back up for almost an hour

This list could go on and on, but the point is that those rough days and tedious moments happen to all of us, and some days it feels like the last straw—like if you see one more high number on your meter you might just fall apart. Some days you just want to scream at the idea of counting one more plate of carbohydrates, stabbing your body with one more syringe, or having to listen to one more ignorant relative lecture you on how a diabetic is *supposed* to eat.

Those days happen. And sure, it'd be great if we could all suck it up and say to ourselves, "Oh, don't worry about it. Life is beautiful, the sun is shining, and tomorrow is a brand new day!" But in reality, that's not really easy to think or say in the moment of a Bad Day for Diabetes. And that's okay—you don't actually have to become a diabetic Mr. Rogers.

Have you ever looked those Bad Days for Diabetes right in the eyes and said, "Wow, you are truly screwing up my day! This day would be so much better without you! I am so frustrated I could hurl this glucose meter out the window!"

Can you recall the last time you experienced *one of those days* with diabetes where your blood sugar was either too high or too low? Where you struggled with every decision around food? Where everything went in exactly the opposite direction that you needed it to?

In five words, describe how those days feel:

1. _____

2. _____

3. _____

4. _____

5. _____

They're different than burnout. Those days don't last. Regardless, those are the days when we've gotta brush ourselves off and stand back up when we're ready.

On the other hand, maybe it's not *just* a bad day ... maybe it's something bigger? In fact, it's good to realize that there is more going on beyond the surface, beyond the day-to-day weight of diabetes. Uncovering all of that can be scary or intimidating or overwhelming, but in order to move beyond your burnout, acknowledging those overwhelming struggles needs to happen. And that is called "digging deeper."

Digging Deeper

Instead of just experiencing a "bad day" where everything seems to be working against you for a day or two, or general exhaustion of the daily responsibilities of diabetes management, your burnout might be part of a much deeper struggle.

Here's what digging deeper looks like from clients I've worked with in my coaching practice (all names and identifying characteristics have been changed to protect privacy):

JANE: Jane feels constantly frustrated because of the pressure from all around her to eat a low-carbohydrate diet. She expresses her frustration by bingeing on carbohydrates almost every night of the week when no one is around, after trying to be "perfect" all day long. On the outside, Jane feels as if she doesn't have any willpower and that she's a "bad diabetic" because she doesn't eat like a diabetic should.

Digging Deeper: After asking Jane what's really going on in her head, it turns out that the constant pressure to eat a healthy diet has led Jane to feeling as if everything is off-limits. She winds up practically starving herself, eating only veggies and yogurt for most of the day. By the time she gets home, she's desperately hungry and binges, which only encourages the habit of thinking she's a failure.

The real issue is not Jane's inability to eat perfectly. Instead, Jane's focus will be about evolving her perspective on what she's "allowed" to eat and learning how to treat her body with compassion around food.

DAN: Dan's burnout is the result of feeling caught in a pattern of blaming himself for having a high A1C, and he feels as if nothing he does makes a difference. He sees himself as a failure and figures he'll never do it perfectly, so he might as well stop trying.

Digging Deeper: It turns out that Dan has actually set himself up for failure by expecting too much improvement too soon. He sets very unrealistic goals for himself and gets quickly discouraged when he can't meet them. He feels so stuck in the trenches that he has no idea where to start making improvements and is constantly beating himself up for it.

The real issue is not Dan's inability to become perfect overnight. Instead, Dan's focus will be on learning how to create smaller, realistic, achievable changes and goals with plenty of room to make mistakes along the way.

ALEX: Alex has been avoiding checking his blood sugar and ignoring the symptoms of hyperglycemia and ketosis for a very long time—years, actually. Every now and then, he says to himself "C'mon, Alex! Start checking your blood sugar more often!" and he sets out with new intentions of checking his blood sugar every day, only to be faced with a mental block and the same old habit of avoiding it.

Digging Deeper: In reality, Alex is very capable of checking his blood sugar but he's convinced himself that he doesn't actually deserve to be healthier. He blames himself for where he is and has developed a tremendous fear of trying to make things better but possibly failing. He feels safer when he doesn't try at all and knows there's no risk of further disappointment. In fact, he even admitted that his father often expresses his disappointment that Alex didn't get into an Ivy League college, like he did, and never became a doctor. That disappointment and shame has flooded many areas of Alex's own self-worth.

While Alex does certainly need to start checking his blood sugar more often, the real issue is his own self-worth, not his ability to prick his finger a few times a day. Starting here, how he views his own life, must be the real focus.

SARAH: Sarah has not exercised in four years, she's gaining weight, and she isn't making oh-so-great choices around food. (And yes, her blood sugar is higher, too.) The worst part is that she *used* to be in awesome shape, and compared to four years ago, when making time for running was easy, Sarah now has two very young kids who keep her very busy. She knows that if she starts exercising again, she'll naturally start eating better, too, but the idea of exercising again is so overwhelming. She knows she's out of shape, and she has tried to go running in the past few years but it hurts so much and is so hard that she feels defeated and depressed, giving up almost instantly.

Digging Deeper: Sarah is holding herself to a standard that worked for her life four years ago, not today. Instead of easing into exercise after two pregnancies, four years without running, and her new role as a mother, she's setting very unrealistic goals for herself, doomed for failure. Learning to acknowledge her new responsibilities and how to create much more reasonable goals around both her exercise and her schedule will help Sarah give herself room to succeed.

JACK: Jack was diagnosed with diabetes a long time ago, and for a very long time he has been an "awesome-almost-perfect-diabetic." Even to this day, he checks his blood sugar six times a day, takes his insulin, counts his carbs, and exercises. But Jack is tired. He doesn't show it in his actions, but he definitely feels tired and even a little angry. Angry that he has to deal with this every day for the rest of his life without any vacations.

Digging Deeper: Jack has gotten so good at being as close to "perfect" as possible in his diabetes, that he doesn't know how to step back and give himself a little bit of space to relax. Maybe that means deciding to rest on the couch and watch movies for an entire weekend instead of exercising. Maybe that even means eating a lot of junk food that weekend while managing his blood sugar a bit less carefully than he usually does. Jack will learn how to give himself the freedom to be imperfect and slack-off for a weekend without feeling guilty. Instead, he'll acknowledge how hard he works on a daily basis for his health and that taking two days "off" is okay and well-deserved.

The stories above illustrate that while your literal actions are symptoms of diabetes burnout, the real cause of your burnout can be much bigger or deeper than simply feeling sick of life with diabetes. Acknowledging the deeper story behind your burnout is the key to know where to begin when you aim to *overcome* your burnout.

Now, it's your turn.

What are the literal actions or behaviors of your burnout? Be sure to include the specifics of your burnout behavior, the length of time your burnout has persisted, and any possible event that might have triggered your burnout.

Example: I've hardly checked my blood sugar in the last six months, ever since my last doctor's appointment.

_____

_____

_____

_____

_____

_____

_____

_____

_____

_____

Digging deeper, what do you feel is truly driving your emotional and mental burnout?

Example: I felt like such a failure at my last doctor's appointment because of my high A1C. I'm just so tired of trying to do better and always failing. I have no idea how to get back on track. And I've developed a really good habit of telling myself I just suck at diabetes management.

_____

_____

_____

_____

_____

_____

_____

Is there a particular aspect of your life outside of diabetes that you feel is feeding your burnout?

Example: As a kid, my parents often scolded me for not getting perfect grades in school. I feel like my choices are perfection and failure, and there's no other option.

_____

_____

_____

_____

_____

_____

_____

_____

_____

What is one thing you believe would give you more of the support you need in order to face the challenges of diabetes management every day?

Example: Maybe a friend, who lives with diabetes, who is also struggling but working on improving. We could set goals together and keep each other from putting too much pressure on ourselves to be perfect.

_____

_____

_____

_____

_____

_____

_____

_____

Depression or Burnout: What's the Difference?

There's no denying that living with diabetes puts us at a higher risk for developing depression. Dr. Jen Nash, a psychologist who also lives with type 1 diabetes, explains that we are actually two to three times *more* likely to experience depression compared to our nondiabetic friends and family.

"The diabetes–depression link is bidirectional," explains Dr. Nash, "meaning that not only do those living with diabetes often manifest depression; but people with depression are more vulnerable to the development of type 2 diabetes. Although research has attempted to understand if depression increases the risk of type 1 diabetes, it is still unclear, with studies yielding very mixed results."

In addition to those whose families have a history of depression or clear chemical imbalance that could be helped with proper medications, Dr. Nash adds that some psychologists connect depression in people with diabetes as a reaction to the loss of their once nondiabetic life and body.

"Depression can also be a mask for anger," says Dr. Nash, "but it is often viewed as a socially unacceptable emotion to express. Depression can mask anger towards diabetes, concentrating the bad feelings towards diabetes at the self."

So what does *depression* look like? While diabetes burnout behavior and symptoms revolve specifically around diabetes management, *depression* affects your behavior in many or most parts of your life.

Dr. Nash shares several symptoms to look for:

Thinking

- Inability to concentrate
- Inability to make decisions
- Loss of interest in the things going on around you, and in other people
- Self-criticism: I've made a mess of everything
- Self-blame: It's all my fault
- Self-loathing: I'm utterly useless
- Activities seem pointless
- Pessimism: This will never change; there's nothing I can do
- Preoccupation with problems, failures, and bad feelings
- Believing you deserve to be punished
- Thinking about harming yourself

Feelings

- Sadness, misery, unhappiness
- Feeling overwhelmed by everyday demands; feeling burdened
- Low confidence and poor self-esteem

- Loss of pleasure, satisfaction, and enjoyment
- Apathy, numbness
- Feeling disappointed, discouraged, or hopeless
- Feeling unattractive or ugly
- Helplessness
- Irritability, tension, anxiety, and worry
- Guilt

Behavior

- Reduced activity levels; doing less than usual
- Everything feels like an effort
- Difficulty getting out of bed in the morning
- Withdrawal—from people, work, relaxations, or pleasures
- Bouts of restlessness
- Sighing, groaning, crying

Bodily Changes

- Loss of appetite or increased appetite
- Disturbed sleep, especially waking early in the morning
- Loss of interest in sex
- Fatigue, lack of energy, or exhaustion
- Inertia: inability to get going, dragging oneself around

If you think you're experiencing depression rather than burnout, you can start by turning to a trustworthy friend or family member who can support you while you research the best resources in your area for help. Whether it be a therapist, psychologist, psychiatrist, or another form of support altogether, taking those steps to getting the help you need is worth your while! Dr. Nash shares some hopeful insight: "The good news is that depression and diabetes-related burnout are treatable and many people go on to make a full recovery. The other good news (although it might be little comfort if you are in the midst of dealing with depression right now) is that many people who recover from depression report that the experience deepened their self-knowledge and understanding of life."

How Burnout Can Impact Other Areas of Life

Sure, the most obvious area of your life that is affected by diabetes burnout is *your diabetes*, but other parts of your life may feel the weight of it, too. Actually, even just day-to-day diabetes management can impact other areas of your life, right? Acknowledging the impact your burnout has on other parts of your life is crucial because it can help you see just how destructive one of your current habits around diabetes may be to other parts, people, or goals in your life. That realization can serve as a great motivator! If you're able to connect your burnout to your lack of progress at work, you may find you're that much more inspired to address your diabetes struggles for the sake of your goals at work. Finding inspiration for your diabetes *outside* of your diabetes is never a bad thing!

Secondly, if your burnout or a habit around your diabetes is negatively impacting the way you treat or behave around the people in your life, that's important to acknowledge for the sake of your relationships and the people who care about you.

For example, when my fiance and I first started dating, he really didn't know anything about type 1 diabetes. During one of our very first arguments as a couple, I realized I was having a low blood sugar. I remember trying to say, "Roger, I can't do this right now, my blood sugar's low." Except ... that's not really how it sounded when it was coming out of my mouth, because I was *so low*, and it was smooshed into whatever we were also arguing about at the time. Frustrated with my inability to communicate logically, he said, "You're not making any sense!" and kept trying to defend his stance in our original argument. "I'm lowwwwww!" I finally yelled. (Then he got me a juice box.) Ever since, he's able to notice when my blood sugar is low much more quickly and knows that trying to communicate with me about anything important during those moments isn't a good idea.

When you add *burnout* to the regular list of diabetes responsibilities and mix it all in with your day-to-day life and relationships, things can get pretty stressful.

Here are a few areas of life that can be impacted by your personal diabetes burnout:

- **Family relationships and overall stress in the home:** Does stress around your diabetes cause arguments and stress throughout the entire home? Just as we feel anxiety and worry when a loved one is in the hospital, our family members may feel constant worry and stress over their inability to successfully help us with our diabetes burnout.

- **Friendships and socialization:** Do your blood sugars impact your energy and your mood so extensively that it shows up in how you relate to your friends? Do you regularly hide your diabetes from your friends and have more high blood sugars as a result?
- **Dating and new relationships:** Does diabetes burnout keep new people in your life from getting to know the real you? If you're hiding diabetes from a potential new relationship, will this limit how well someone can truly be able to know about you and your life?
- **Long-term relationships and marriage:** Are your blood sugars a source of constant stress or frustration in your relationship? How much worry does your partner carry daily over your diabetes?
- **Education (grades K–12, college, etc.):** There's no denying that out-of-whack blood sugars impact our ability to focus, remember, and learn. Is your burnout impacting your grades, enthusiasm, and attendance for school?
- **Work and career:** Similar to school, your work and career goals probably require a great deal of energy, which can be easily limited by diabetes burnout that includes higher blood sugars. Additionally, are you often calling in sick because of diabetes-related issues?
- **Life goals and aspirations:** What do you dream of accomplishing one day? Whether it's starting your own business, having a child, running a marathon, or writing a book, your burnout can get in the way of your dreams.

Okay, now it's your turn.

How has diabetes and burnout impacted other areas of *your* life?

_____

_____

_____

_____

_____

_____

_____

_____

_____

You might even try talking to the people involved in those situations above, asking them how *they* feel your burnout has impacted their life. You might be surprised to realize they worry more than you thought, or that they've noticed changes in your personality and energy you didn't realize were noticeable.

Habits That Never Have and Never Will Help

A funny thing we all tend to do in many areas of life—diabetic or not—is try the same methods over and over and over, even though they never really lead to the success we're looking for. You know that Albert Einstein quote? "Insanity is doing the same thing over and over and expecting a different result?" Well, it's quite possible the man knew somebody living with diabetes 'cause he's got a really great point!

A classic example of this "over and over" approach is picking a new fad diet, following it obsessively for a week while also obsessively trying to make it to the gym every single day … and then *kersplat* everything goes out the window because that strict diet and pressure to exercise every day was too much to maintain. And yet, in a few months, you might try to do the same thing all over again. You might've pointed the finger at yourself, blaming yourself for not being able to stick to it or follow through when the real issue is simply that habit of asking too much of yourself all at once.

Instead, developing the ability to step back and see what wasn't working—rather than blaming yourself—is the trick to creating a new plan that *will* lead you to your goal.

When it comes to your burnout or diabetes as a whole, you've probably developed a few habits in how you attempt to pull out of your burnout, become the perfect diabetic overnight, or suddenly eat a diet of leafy greens, cauliflower, and Brussels sprouts in an attempt to lose weight.

Let's take a look at what others have to say about those habits that never seem to help. The following are anonymous statements gathered through a survey from people of all ages with type 1 and type 2 diabetes:

The habits we have that never seem to help...

"I keep trying to love salad. I mean, I do, but it just doesn't compare to a cheeseburger. I'll go a week or so making delicious salads and then I remember how much tastier bread is!"

❧

"Around exercise? Often. Often. Often. All throughout my life. There was a period early in my 40s where I was going to the gym and got into decent shape. I've always been slender so it's easy to trick myself that I'm in good shape. I tried sports when I was younger and just couldn't do it. I always wanted to be an awesome athlete, to no avail. Now I'm almost 50 and my chance is over. Makes me sad."

❧

"I try to eat low-carb every now and then, but I never make it very long, because it's just too hard to do it perfectly! I breakdown after a few days and eat every carb in sight."

❧

"I always say I'm going to start running every day and mentally I'm totally up for it, but then my sugars are high or low and I feel too tired to do it. Or I go for a few days and end up going so low that I have to stop because I'm spending a fortune on sugar and feel like utter crap. Not being able to do something you want to do is the worst feeling in the world and it's so frustrating."

❧

"I used to do this, stop and start over and over with exercise, but now I have found I have to plan to change up what I am doing every month in order to not quit exercising in general."

(continued)

(continued)

The habits we have that never seem to help…

"I tell myself I'm gonna check my blood sugar six times a day, measure my insulin doses really perfectly … but as soon as I think about having to check six times a day, every day, I get overwhelmed and give up. I do it to myself."

∾

"I have this image in my head of how I'm supposed to be, and I create a crazy intimidating plan to be that person, and I fail like crazy within just a few days. Over and over and over. Between all the attempts to be that person, I beat myself up for not being able to do it."

∾

"I'll go to the gym and work out like three or four times, but then as soon as I take more than two days off, I feel really guilty and I stop going altogether. I know it's dumb, because I could just go again on day 3, but I just have it stuck in my head that I have to go at least every other day. It's so dumb."

∾

"I have read so many diet books! So many workout plans! I've done them all! But I've only done them for like two weeks at a time, because I go all-in, head-first, hardcore, and burn out so fast. I've done this so many times, I've lost count. But damn, I sure do know a lot about dieting and exercise … just not how to actually make it work for my life!"

∾

"Logging on paper for my endocrinologist. I can't ever keep up with it. I know that knowing how many carbs I intake, what foods I eat, and how much insulin I take, in addition to the blood sugars numbers provided by my CGM would help exponentially, but it's just too much work to do for any length of time."

(continued)

(continued)

The habits we have that never seem to help...

"The plan or habit I have is to count my carbs more efficiently. This doesn't work well for me because of my gastroparesis. I never know when food is going to digest so I am constantly battling highs and lows for no known reason because food is either not getting into my system or it's digesting from four weeks ago. It is really frustrating."

∾

"Every time I try to eat better, I don't eat enough. I end up so freaking hungry and starving that I binge after, like, a week. I've done this so many times! I need to learn how to eat healthier without starving myself at the same time! I know I'm not doing it right, I know."

∾

"I try to end my addiction with the white foods—potatoes, rice, bread, pasta—and cut them out completely rather than just reducing how much I eat them. I always stick to it for maybe a week or two, then I just can't stand it anymore and go back to eating them."

∾

"I tend to start a new exercise routine in the fall (when it's cooler, and I won't kill myself in the heat of summer), but then it gets too cold so I slack off in the winter, try again in the spring, then fall off the wagon again in the summer."

Coping Skills: Helpful or Not-So-Helpful?

At first glance, the word "coping" seems like a quick way to say you're just dealing with what is dealt your way, but if you've been engaged in some type of burnout behavior for several years, there may be a deeper but very subtle reason why holding on to your burnout feels better than moving forward. It's hard to believe we would continue doing something that we know is sabotaging our own life or holding us back from achieving our goals. Deep down, no matter how destructive the behavior might be, there is probably a "benefit" to that behavior that helps you "cope" with something else going on.

Imagine that you or someone you know has a habit of dating people who treat you poorly. Even though you know you're being treated poorly you continue to let those people into your life, reinforcing your own belief that you don't deserve to be loved or treated with respect. Despite the obvious negative aspects of this habit, being treated poorly and continuing to believe that you deserve to be treated that way may feel like the easiest path to continue on because it's familiar to you. Standing up for yourself and realizing your own self-worth can actually seem like the more difficult and scary path, simply because it isn't what you're used to.

While that example may seem a bit extreme or hard to believe for someone who is in a loving relationship, it's very common, and the same type of logic can explain some forms of purposeful neglect around diabetes management.

From a distance, bingeing on food at the end of a stressful day may seem like a habit that is just really hard to break because you don't have enough "willpower," but if we dig deeper into that habit we might discover that abusing yourself with food actually serves as a protective reinforcement for a personal belief.

For some, bingeing on food can be a simple method of self-sabotage and a self-fulfilling prophecy: "I don't deserve to feel good about myself, I suck at managing my diabetes, and I don't deserve to treat my body with respect."

Well, sure, who wouldn't have a hard time managing their blood sugars if they were abusing food every night? I certainly would have a hard time, too! But if a person is so used to that protective shield of feeling ashamed of themselves for their behavior, then that habit of abusing food feels safe and familiar rather than self-destructive and detrimental to their overall well-being.

Denial is another form of coping that could easily be mistaken for the actual problem. If you asked 10 people in denial about their diabetes *why* they were in denial, each answer would be different. Instead of seeing denial as the problem, let's think of it merely as the symptom of an emotional struggle or form of burnout in life with diabetes.

For example:

- *"I'm totally scared because my entire family has passed away from diabetes complications and it's like I'm frozen with fear about my future. I watched my mom, brother and my uncle lose their feet. I'm terrified, so I do nothing."*
- *"I hate blood. I'm terrified of needles and the idea of poking my finger several times a day. No way. I can't do it. I will literally lose my mind and break down if I have to look at my own blood every day."*
- *"I feel like such a failure for getting diabetes in the first place, I can't face it. I feel so guilty. So worthless. I did this to myself and I deserve it and that's that. I don't believe there's anything I can do about it."*
- *"I hate diabetes and everything about it. It's so unfair that I have to deal with this and no one else in my family has it. It interrupts everything, and who in the world wants to count carbs and take shots all day? I'm 16, I want to be a normal teenager. So I'm just not gonna deal with my stupid diabetes."*
- *"I. Just. Can't. I've never been good at dieting, exercising, and I've been an emotional eater since I was a little girl. Always overweight. Now I have to be perfect because a doctor told me I have diabetes? I can't. I've struggled with these things my whole life, and I gave up a long time ago."*

The stories above are *not* simply stories about coping, they're stories about fear, phobia, panic attacks, self-esteem, anger, helplessness, and hopelessness. Denial is just what those stories look like on the outside when the people in those stories stopped taking care of their diabetes. But the road to "reality" will be very different for each person.

The "benefits" can also be very subtle. For instance, avoiding checking your blood sugar because you're sick of living with diabetes may also be your way of continuing to feel like a victim rather than someone who stands up and takes charge and faces challenges with pride. Despite the benefits of facing a challenge in life with pride, being the victim may simply be what you're used to, and therefore, it feels safer and easier to do—even though it doesn't make you happy.

Sometimes, becoming the person you truly aspire to be, like someone who treats their body with respect around food or is empowered by their own diabetes and other challenges in life, can be far scarier and more overwhelming than sticking with the behavior you're most familiar with, even if it's hurting you in the long-run and causing a great deal of unhappiness.

What are the "benefits" of your burnout behavior? How does continuing any self-destructive habits reinforce negative beliefs you may have about yourself or continue to help you avoid other things in your life?

Example: Bingeing on food late at night, which sabotages my blood sugars, helps me continue to avoid admitting how lonely I feel and how insecure I feel about meeting new people.

_____

_____

_____

_____

_____

_____

_____

_____

_____

Now imagine what it would be like to let go of that behavior that serves as a protective shield for something else or the personal belief about yourself that keeps you trapped in your burnout. What would it be like if you *let go* of that familiar behavior and let yourself become the version of yourself that you've always aspired to be?

Example: If I stopped bingeing on food to purposefully sabotage my health and confidence, I would have to admit I'm lonely and make an effort to go meet new people, start taking care of myself, and embrace all the great things about who I am that other people might like about me, too.

So what do helpful or healthy coping skills look like? A truly positive form of coping would allow you to both express and acknowledge whatever you're struggling with *and* it would help you take on those emotions in a way that wasn't also self-destructive, but instead, was supportive of your goals around your health and life with diabetes.

While going for a run, practicing yoga, or playing a game of chess may be some of the specific hobbies in your life that help you set aside your woes and relax, in the end, the way you truly cope in any given moment will come down to the thoughts you put into your very own head.

And those thoughts reside in your Mental Skills Toolbox. Looking at what is currently sitting in that toolbox (the not-so-helpful coping skills) is a crucial part of digging deeper, followed by thinking about what kinds of tools you'd like to keep in that toolbox instead.

Inside Your Mental Skills Toolbox

Whether we're failing or succeeding, the way we think about our diabetes and the messages we tell ourselves about our own ability to manage this disease determines whether we beat ourselves up for feeling burned-out or we give ourselves the compassion and understanding we deserve. The mental tools we use can help us take on any emotion we face in life with diabetes.

If Superman had been constantly told his powers were creepy and freaky, instead of awesome and impressive, then he would've grown up being ashamed of what he was capable of. If you constantly tell yourself that you're a failure because you can't manage your diabetes perfectly, you will continue to feel ashamed of yourself. The messages in your head absolutely lead to how you feel and what you believe about who you are.

Without having ever met you, I already know that if you're living with diabetes every day, you are a courageous person. I already know you have an admirable level of strength and persistence. I am already impressed by your ability to get out of bed every morning and take on this disease, even on the days when you make mistakes or feel really burned-out and barely make an effort.

But if you are stuck in a pattern of shaming yourself for being imperfect, frustrated, and exhausted in diabetes management, then it's only expected that the pattern of burnout will continue, too.

One of the most important tools in your Mental Skills Toolbox for managing your own burnout is how you think about the reality of your diabetes and your ability to take care of it.

Imagine for a moment that you own a 100-pound goldendoodle who has more energy than a caffeinated toddler, and he loves the mud. In my real life, that goldendoodle's name is Blue. Despite being part poodle, which is thought of as prissy and proper, Blue is often referred to as a "dumpster dog" because of his uncontrollable need to eat garbage and roll around in the mud. Every puddle of mud wants to party with my dog. The result? There are constantly dirty dog prints on the nice hardwood floors of my home.

When Blue came into my life as my very first puppy, his mud-season dirtiness drove me nuts. I was constantly mopping and sweeping the floors, constantly giving him impromptu baths, and getting frustrated with Blue for hitting up every muddy area of the backyard.

As I think about it from a distance, it sounds like an incredible waste of energy: getting frustrated because Blue just couldn't help but be a dog and roll around in the mud. And this reminds me of diabetes burnout.

It's simply a fact that there will be times in my life when I just don't have the energy and motivation I need to keep up with my diabetes as well as I'd like to. I know there will be a couple of months each year when I might eat more carbohydrates than I know I should, or a few days when I barely check my blood sugar two times a day, because I'm just flippin' tired of pricking my fingers. And I also know that each spring, my dog Blue is going to roll around in the mud and create a disaster that I will need to clean up.

Today, not only do I anticipate and expect a muddy goldendoodle and muddy floors, I appreciate that his boundless, carefree spirit is what makes him Blue (and what makes him muddy). In my diabetes, not only do I anticipate and expect that those days, weeks, or months of burnout will happen, I also understand that part of what makes me human is my inability to be a perfect diabetic robot. And that's okay. (Besides, perfection is so boring!)

How do you currently talk to yourself about your diabetes? Write down some of the exact thoughts you have on a daily basis about your personal ability to manage your diabetes.

Example: I feel like a bad diabetic, and I suck at managing my diabetes!

_____

_____

_____

_____

_____

_____

_____

_____

_____

Look at the statements you listed above and circle all of the statements that encourage the belief that you can't handle diabetes, that you're doing a lousy job, that you're not as perfect as you "should" be.

Now read those statements to yourself, but this time, put yourself in the mind of the most compassionate person you've ever met; it can be someone you made up in your imagination or maybe it's your loving Aunt Gloria who smells like old furniture and pistachio nuts, but she thinks you're incredible and deserve all good things. As you re-read those statements, ask that compassionate voice what you really need.

More blaming and scolding? Or do you need something more? Like:

- A really big diabetes hug
- Understanding, because this diabetes thing is *hard work*
- Freedom to make mistakes
- Forgiveness for making mistakes
- Help from a professional mental health therapist for stress or anxiety
- Help from a certified diabetes educator
- A support group filled with other people who know what it's like
- A voice that says, "It's okay, you don't have to be perfect. Let's try again."
- A new goal that *doesn't* involve total perfection
- A new goal that focuses on one specific and simple detail of diabetes management
- A new way of thinking about your ability to manage your diabetes that doesn't require you to be perfect, blame you for mistakes, and offers plenty of compassion for the immensity of this disease

Now, imagine what kinds of thoughts that compassionate person would think about your ability to manage your diabetes. Imagine what kinds of repeated thoughts that person would put into *your* head over and over when you're facing the daily responsibilities, worries, stress, and frustration of diabetes. Even if you don't believe them right this very moment, or even if they aren't remotely close to being a natural thought you'd easily keep in your head at this moment, write down what the most compassionate person you know would say to you when you're overwhelmed by diabetes:

Example: You are facing something tremendous every day. Take a deep breath. Keep going.

_____

_____

_____

_____

_____

_____

_____

_____

In time, maybe they'll evolve, maybe they'll stay the same, or maybe they'll simply get mixed in with some of the less compassionate thoughts you might currently hold onto today. This is a process. A gradual transition—that starts with practice—to a point in your life where your head is so filled with support and compassion that there isn't nearly as much room for the voice that shames you and blames you for your diabetes imperfections.

Resilience: The One Thing You Can't Get a Prescription For! (That you definitely need in your Mental Skills Toolbox!)

By Leann Harris
www.delphidiabetescoaching.com

I really think they are missing one vital piece when writing prescriptions for diabetes supplies. Yes, we need a glucometer, test strips, pills, possibly needles, and insulin. Don't forget lancets, alcohol wipes, and glucagon.

Why doesn't anyone ever write out a prescription for resilience?

Resilience sounds like it would be a very powerful, fancy drug if it ever hit the market. "Wow, how did you lose all that weight?" "Well, I started taking Resilience and it works wonders!" Lucky for us, this drug is much cheaper on the street than anything you could buy.

We've already proven we have some dose of resilience in us by the fact that we're still breathing. Our bodies are (mostly) still functioning. While we may feel anger and sorrow, we keep breathing, if nothing else.

Let me explain a bit about resilience. When I use it, I'm not talking about "putting up with something," "tolerating," or "in spite of." Those feelings imply "suppression" or "disengagement." To me, those words have the ring of a problem that persists constantly for us, and which we heavily plod our way through to get to the end of each day, with no significant resolution to the problem or change in our circumstances.

Resilience implies a sense of groundedness or connectedness with our inner capacities. It's having a clear view of reality in front of us and what resources we have to work with it. Resilience is when you've taken stock of what you have to work with, weighed what's most appropriate to the situation, and that wisdom is employed to use the right tool. By fully recognizing the problem at hand, we are

(continued)

(continued)

Resilience: The One Thing You Can't Get a Prescription For! (That you definitely need in your Mental Skills Toolbox!)

By Leann Harris
www.delphidiabetescoaching.com

able to address it, to root out its cause, and to engage it. In doing so, we explore undiscovered places within ourselves that can only benefit us if we can learn to navigate them. Personal resilience comes into play when we are curious about what we truly need in the moment, whether it's comfort, safety, appreciation or acknowledgement of all of our hard work. We no longer want to ignore or brush off pieces of our lives, but want to find a way to make everything fit and run smoothly.

Diabetes can seem like the most demanding challenge on earth. But with resilience, we can look at it afresh each time. Maybe we've been trying to get over feeling depressed, but just can't seem to shake it. We've talked to friends, we've read books, we've done everything we think we should do, but we still don't seem to feel any better. We have gone through the list and nothing has worked. What if we were curious about what we're really feeling? What if we tried to really feel what this distress is all about? What if we weren't so quick to label and dismiss our feelings? Labeling ourselves "depressed" doesn't help us.

Here are a few questions to dig deeper:

- Has it helped us to struggle against being depressed?
- What are our fears and concerns in this situation?
- Could we stop trying to *not* feel upset, even for five minutes?
- How many times a day do you struggle against the way you feel? How many times a day has struggling worked for you?
- Could it possibly be that the only action needed is for us to stop struggling?

Part of resilience is realizing we'll feel something, but we can make another choice, regardless. We may feel uncomfortable being depressed, but trying all sorts of exercises to feel better

(continued)

(continued)

Resilience: The One Thing You Can't Get a Prescription For! (That you definitely need in your Mental Skills Toolbox!)

By Leann Harris
www.delphidiabetescoaching.com

isn't helping any. One option is to not keep trying to manipulate life. Yes, it will feel uncomfortable, but so does something that isn't working. What if you were no longer focused on stopping the depression, but instead focused on what you can do right now?

Take a sheet of paper, and copy down your answers. On a scale of 1 through 10, with 1 being *Forget it* to 10 being *I'll give it 100 percent,* how willing are you to do the following:

- How willing are you to cry or grieve?
- How willing are you listen to what you're telling yourself about being depressed, even if it's hard to catch the thoughts?
- How flexible are you being? How willing are you to try new things?
- How nonjudgmental are you being with the world? With yourself?
- How open are you being to life?
- How uncomfortable and fearful are you willing to admit out loud? To yourself?
- Could you really listen to what you are feeling, deep inside?
- Are you willing to feel the way you feel, and take a single step, regardless of your present feelings?
- Would you be willing to name something you've always wanted to do, but never thought you'd be up to trying? How much do you think you'll lose if you were to try it?
- How willing are you to take up a hobby you used to enjoy, no matter what emotion you're feeling in the moment?

Willingness is sometimes called active acceptance. It helps to think of it as embracing the fact that it's part of your life so that it is no longer blocking you from moving forward. So you may choose to go out with friends, even if it's not an ideal situation for you. You may choose to take up painting again, even if you don't feel like your

(continued)

(*continued*)

Resilience: The One Thing You Can't Get a Prescription For! (That you definitely need in your Mental Skills Toolbox!)

By Leann Harris
www.delphidiabetescoaching.com

best self. Active acceptance is a moment-by-moment choice, and every choice we make is an act of resilience.

Resilience is a powerful tool in our diabetes-coping arsenal. Curiosity about the edges of what we're experiencing can be the fuel we need to stay resilient. Out of all the questions I ask myself, my most useful is, "Yes, that is so, *and* what else?" What other possibilities are there that I just haven't explored yet? How willing am I to even look? How open can I be to the answers? How much energy can I save by accepting the card I've been dealt? How much am I willing to lose by fighting what is, and when is enough going to be enough?

Knowing Where You Are ... and Where You Want to Go

At this point, you spent the past two chapters looking closely at emotions you feel in relation to diabetes, your specific actions and behaviors surrounding diabetes management, and the way you talk to yourself whether you're thriving or struggling. Honest, intense reflection.

The next step? Determining exactly what you'd like to focus on and exactly what you'd like to accomplish. But creating realistic goals around blood sugars, nutrition, and exercise isn't always easy. Many of us create goals that are practically impossible to accomplish, or expectations that set us up for absolute failure. Sometimes we create goals that are doable, but we don't tend to give ourselves enough time to actually *do* them! And last but not least, sometimes our goals simply are not clear enough.

The next chapter is going to help you create specific and logical goals for any aspect of life with diabetes.

I Want to Be Perfect by Tomorrow (or I'm Giving Up)!

3

Setting Yourself Up for Success with Realistic Goals and Fewer Pitfalls

Have you ever decided you're suddenly going to do everything you're "supposed to do" in diabetes management—like counting carbohydrates, taking your medications and insulin whenever you're supposed to, checking your blood sugar at least four times a day, and, of course, avoiding any foods that are sweet and delicious and "bad for diabetics"—only to find yourself frustrated and off-the-wagon barely a few days later?

Chances are, if you're like most of us, those ambitious efforts to jump out of your burnout and jump right into diabetic perfection don't last long—because it's just *too overwhelming*. Or maybe you haven't gotten to that point of setting new goals of perfection because you're not even sure where to start and it all feels … well, again, too overwhelming.

Whether you've tried to be perfect or you haven't tried at all, the problem is often the same: the diabetes to-do list can feel so tremendously daunting and very few of us can really handle that pressure to be perfect.

But if you aren't aiming for perfection, then where do you aim?

This chapter is about setting yourself up for success through learning how to set goals concerning your life with diabetes that are not only realistic but also very clear and specific. At the risk of abusing the words "realistic" and "achievable" in this chapter, I'm going to use the word "awesome" much more often instead.

Developing the ability to create really awesome goals for any part of your life, related to your diabetes or not, is one of the most valuable skills you may ever develop. Too often, many of us have a tendency to make giant, lofty, vague, impossible goals that only wind up making us feel like failures when we don't follow through and achieve them. Let's change that!

Have you ever had a doctor's appointment that went something like this:

Doctor: *You need to start taking better care of your diabetes.*

Patient with Diabetes: *Um, yes, I know. I know.*

Doctor: *You need to eat better foods, check your blood sugar four times a day, and exercise at least 150 minutes per week.*

Patient with Diabetes: *Um … okay. Okay.*

Doctor: *Okay, good. I'll see you in six months.*

The problem with this entire scene, whether it happens between you and yourself, your health care team, or a family member, is that it is absolutely setting you up for failure.

One of the most important parts of getting beyond your burnout is about rebuilding confidence in your ability to face diabetes every day, and that's not going to happen if your choices are perfection or failure. Instead, building that confidence can start from creating a challenge you can clearly achieve that will fill you with a feeling of true success. That feeling of success, even from something seemingly very small, is like the gasoline that fuels the engine of a car for someone who is overwhelmed by frustration, lack of confidence, and a habit of negative thinking concerning their own ability to take care of their diabetes.

Take a moment, right now, to close your eyes and envision a version of you who is proud of yourself for facing diabetes each day, and giving your best, even when your best isn't perfect. Seriously. Put down the book for a moment or two and envision that version of yourself.

Okay?

That version of yourself is somewhere beneath the burnout. Instead of scolding yourself for imperfections and frustration, that other version of yourself knows that some days your best is nearly perfect and other days your best is a little … wrinkly. That other version of yourself knows that diabetes is challenging, from moment to moment.

Through learning how to set awesome goals as you work toward becoming that version of yourself who is confident and okay with imperfection, I want you to *feel* successful through small steps and small achievements.

Don't Be Pushy … On Yourself!

So, wait a moment. Literally. Right here. If you have this book in your hands then it's safe to assume that at some point in the future you probably do *want* to move through your burnout and feel more positive about your life with diabetes, but that doesn't necessarily mean you have to feel that way or start doing anything about it *this* week or even *next* week.

Sometimes, one of the most important parts of creating change in your life is simply *thinking* about that change for a little while! Usually, we think this only applies to fun things like, "Which college am I going to?" or, "Am I ready to move in with my boyfriend?" or, "Do I really want to take that job promotion?"

But even when we're contemplating going from a situation we know we ought to move out of or away from, such as burnout, taking the time to prepare yourself for that mentally, by literally just *thinking* about it, is crucial.

For example, when I stopped powerlifting in the spring of 2012 because of pain in my leg, lower back, wrists, and elbows, I was so tired of thinking about my athletic nutrition and food in general that I just let all the rules of how to fuel your metabolism go out the window. Instead, I ate when I felt like it. Now, for some of you that might not sound like a big deal, but I used to make sure I was eating every three hours to ensure my muscles had the fuel they needed. Not caring, or going five or even eight hours without eating a meal was liberating. Food and the science of nutrition for athletes had been an intense hobby, you could say, for several years by that point, and my head was just tired. This was my own form of burnout around nutrition. Now that's not to say I wasn't eating mostly very healthy things—in fact, I really relished not having to eat as many calories or as many carbohydrates. I lost quite a bit of weight that came from both fat and muscle, and my A1C actually dropped—but I was doing my share of gluten-free baking on the weekends, too! (It was delicious, believe me.)

It wasn't until a full year later that I actually started being interested in nutrition again, but I didn't dive right in and change how I was eating. Instead, I did a little reading. A little thinking. Started listening to a variety of nutrition podcasts. A little more thinking. More reading. And none of this felt like work, because I hadn't put any expectations on myself to change anything or do anything. Instead, I was just delving back into the world of nutrition and thinking about how I might apply it to my life.

And then, I picked a day. I thought to myself, "Starting in two weeks, I'm going to apply some of the major changes around nutrition I've been educating myself about." Two of those changes included eating primarily organic vegetables and grass-fed meats, and getting back to my once-a-week cheat-day rather than having small treats whenever I felt like it. And two weeks later, I genuinely felt interested in the science of nutrition and applying it to my own life again.

Sometimes, it might just be the wrong time to start working on that change. If you're going through a really stressful event—which might even be part of why you're feeling burned-out on diabetes—then maybe it's okay to just do what you can to get through that stressful time of your life until you can bring your attention and energy back to your diabetes. No matter what the answer is, it's important to remember that *right* now might *not* actually be the right time to work on overcoming diabetes burnout, even if you do continue to read about it.

So, I turn back to you and ask, "Are you ready?"

You can keep reading, of course, even if you aren't ready, but make sure you ask yourself, "When do I actually want to start applying what I read to my life with diabetes?"

If you don't ask yourself that question, you may end up trying to force yourself to "get over" your burnout before you're truly ready. Instead of feeling like a project you chose to focus on, it will feel like a chore. (And yes, I realize diabetes is a chore, but getting over your burnout needs to be *your choice*.) And instead of feeling as if you're taking a powerful and brave step forward, it will feel as if you're dragging your feet along in some tedious task you don't care about.

Ask yourself, more specifically, "When am I ready to apply what I read in this book to my own diabetes burnout?" Then stare at the calendar, or close your eyes and listen to that little voice in your head that takes care of you. That quiet little voice that we sometimes ignore. Maybe the voice will say, "Next week!" or maybe it will say, "I don't know, but you're not ready quite yet."

Either way, it's okay. Right this very second, ask yourself, "When am I ready?" and reflect on the following options:

- I am ready right this very second!
- I will be ready when I finish reading the book.
- I think I just want to skim this. Put it away for a while. Then come back to it in a month.
- I am totally not ready, but my sister bought me this book, so I feel obligated to read it.
- I'll be ready soon. Maybe next week.
- I have no idea when I'll be ready.
- I really hate diabetes and I need more help before I'll be ready.

Or write your own answer:

Okay, so no matter when you're ready, I hope you move to the next section of this book, because being "ready" still involves small steps and careful thought … without any pressure to be perfect by tomorrow!

Creating (and Accomplishing) Really Awesome Goals

If you've ever decided you're going to "test your blood sugar every day" or "never eat junk food again" then you're not alone, but let's take those two classic goals and give them a major makeover. This is a six-step process to creating goals that will help you feel focused and inspired.

1. Understand Where You're Starting from

You actually did the work on this one back in Chapter 2. Rewrite those sentences from page 26 below about what is currently happening (or not happening) in your life with diabetes today:

_____

_____

_____

_____

_____

2. Be Super, Extremely, Incredibly Specific

Pick a very specific aspect of diabetes to focus on—and I mean *really* specific. A few common examples of goal statements related to diabetes management that are too vague and difficult to take action on are:

I want to live a long and healthy life with diabetes.
I want to take better care my diabetes.

Okay, sure, that's a wonderful thing to aim for, but if you don't boil that down to what you need to focus on *right now*, you'll have absolutely no idea where to start from and nothing specific to aim toward each individual day. A "long and healthy life" is also nearly impossible to measure in any short period of time.

If you've been struggling to make checking your blood sugar a bigger priority, then aiming to suddenly check it at least four times a day, every single day, is just too much too soon. Instead, pick *one (maybe two)* times of the day to focus on. Also, let's replace the phrase *"I want"* with *"I will."*

*I will check my blood sugar each day **before lunch**.*
*I will check my blood sugar each night **before bed**.*

Now the goal you're going to focus on accomplishing has an incredibly specific and achievable action. If you said this goal statement out loud to your friends, they would be able to understand exactly what you're going to work on concerning your diabetes.

Now it's your turn. Write down exactly what you want to accomplish:

_____

_____

_____

_____

_____

3. Make Sure You Can Measure Your Progress

Okay, so we know what you literally want to work on and achieve, but for how long will you focus on this goal? When will you stop to assess your progress? How will you know when it's time to expand your goal?

Let's give this goal statement a time frame:

*I will check my blood sugar, before lunch, each day **for two weeks**.*
*I will check my blood sugar each night, before bed, **for the next four days**.*

Now, you're probably thinking, *"Um … aren't I supposed to check my blood sugar every freaking day for the rest of my life?"* Well, sure, in an ideal world you'd jump right to doing it "perfectly," but what's more important is that you ease in gradually to whatever diabetes responsibility you're aiming to accomplish … setting yourself up for success!

Think of it this way: if you can only handle the pressure of doing something "perfectly" for four days before you get burned-out and quit (followed by beating yourself up emotionally in the process for failing to be perfect), doesn't it make more sense to set a less-than-perfect goal and maintain progress in that goal for an unlimited amount of time? I certainly think so. By adding the specificity of "two weeks" or "four days" or any other period of time to your goal, it takes away the pressure of suddenly feeling as if you need to do this perfectly for the rest of your life.

And lastly, it also gives you a very specific period of time to assess your progress, because let's face it: there's a pretty good chance that at some point during the rest of your entire life with diabetes you'll probably forget to check your blood sugar before lunch. (I know there have certainly been a few days when I've forgotten!)

Now it's your turn. Give your goal statement a clear and specific time frame for measuring progress:

_____

_____

_____

_____

_____

4. Ask Yourself Why This Matters to You

Now that you have a clear goal statement about *what* you want to accomplish, which you can take action on and measure your progress toward as you go, there is something you really need to ask yourself: *why in the world does accomplishing this goal matter? Why do you care about improving your life with diabetes?*

If your first answer is, "Because I want to live a long life with diabetes," then it's time to dig a little deeper. Just like your goal statement, this statement needs to be specific, but more importantly, it needs to ignite something in your mind and heart! While you might think that sounds awfully touchy-feely, digging to the true motivation behind your goal is the secret to ignite your energy to move forward.

This is a typical conversation I might have with a diabetes coaching client when we're trying to dig to the "why" of her goal:

> **Ginger:** *Okay, so you want to take better care of your blood sugar, and you're going to start by trying to check each day before lunch for two weeks … but why is this important to you?*
>
> **Jane:** *Because I want to be healthier and live a long time?*
>
> **Ginger:** *Why?*
>
> **Jane:** *Because I don't want to go blind when I'm older or lose my feet.*
>
> **Ginger:** *What do you want instead?*
>
> **Jane:** *I want to feel good about my diabetes and feel healthy.*
>
> **Ginger:** *What else?*
>
> **Jane:** *I don't want to struggle with accepting it.*
>
> **Ginger:** *If you're not struggling to accept it, how do you want to feel about it instead?*
>
> **Jane:** *At peace. I want to feel at peace with my diabetes.*
>
> **Ginger:** *You want to feel at peace with your diabetes?*
>
> **Jane:** *Yes, I want to feel at peace in my life with diabetes.*

That last sentence, "I want to feel at peace in my life with diabetes," touches on a part of Jane's heart and mind that only Jane can truly understand. Whatever that sentence means to her when she envisions it in her mind is her own. It's intangible—a feeling that will be unique to her own experience of diabetes. What "peace" might feel and look like to you and me could be very different to Jane's vision of peace, and that's okay. In fact, that means you've found your *"why"* statement.

Now, it's your turn. Using the following questions as a prompt to help you dig deeper, create the true "why" statement of your goal:

- **How will accomplishing this goal impact your life?**
- **What do you really, really want for your life with diabetes?**

- **Why do you care?**
- **What do you want to feel instead of what you feel now about your diabetes?**
- **Why? Why? Why?**

_____

_____

_____

_____

_____

5. Establish the Tiny, Supportive Details

Think about the habits in your life that have helped to reinforce and perpetuate your burnout. For instance, maybe your blood glucose meter lives in a dark cabinet most of the time, hidden from your sight on a daily basis. Or perhaps even though you live with your parents or your boyfriend or your roommates, nobody in the home ever really talks out loud about your diabetes and therefore it's easier to ignore or feel very alone in living with it. Maybe the ideal time of day when you can go for a walk or a jog outside is the time of day when you usually turn on the TV and become a zombie for an hour. Whatever the habit or situation may be, it needs to be adjusted if we want the outcome to be different.

For example, here are a few ideas to get your mind bubbling:

- Create a safe, visible place in your kitchen where your blood glucose meter is going to live, from now on, whenever you are at home. If you live with a variety of people, then they all need to know about this new adjustment, too.
- Talk out loud about your diabetes at dinnertime with your family, friends, roommates—whomever you eat dinner with! Make it a part of a positive conversation and include those around you who love you.

- Invite your best friend or roommate to walk with you or do a Pilates video together a few days of the week when you might usually zone out in front of the TV.
- Do you have a dog, or maybe your neighbors have a dog you adore and could borrow? Take that little guy for an extra walk and use his energy as a source of motivation for your own goals.
- Pick two days of the week when you will go to the grocery store to get fresh fruits and veggies for the week to help reinforce your goals for healthier nutrition.

While we will dig into nutrition and exercise and diabetes later in the book, the examples above are all about creating *new* habits, *new* routines, that will help reinforce your focus on your goal on any aspect of health or life with diabetes!

And, of course, now it's your turn. Think about a few of the tiny details and habits in life that you can adjust in order to support your diabetes and health:

_____

_____

_____

_____

_____

_____

_____

_____

_____

6. Create a Pick-Up Plan

So what happens if you slip-up and get off-track? Does that mean your goal statement goes out the window and you're back where you started? No way. The creation of any goal statement needs a Pick-Up Plan, too.

Your Pick-Up Plan is for that day or week when everything goes against your goal. When you fall back into old habits or you get so overwhelmed with another part of your life that diabetes goes right out the window. Or maybe it's simply that you hit a few days, a weekend, or even several weeks where you lose sight of your goal, your commitment to your diabetes, and you stop making that goal a priority.

That's okay.

It's okay to get off-track. In fact, if you don't get off-track, fall off the horse, or get derailed at least once on the journey toward your goal, I'd be surprised. In fact, this really only becomes a problem when you confuse getting off-track with failure. Getting off-track happens … and when it's time, you'll get back on-track. *Failing* is when you simply give up completely. Your Pick-Up Plan is for that moment when you're struggling to focus on accomplishing your goal.

The plan needs to help you accomplish three things:

1. Help you acknowledge why you've gotten off-track
2. Support and encourage you with positive self-talk
3. Establish a clear plan for when you will refocus on your goal

Take a look at this example:

Your goal statement: *I will check my blood sugar, before lunch, each day for two weeks.*

Imagine the statement above is the goal you're working on, but after breaking up with your boyfriend or going through a divorce on top of a really stressful project at work, you're really stressed-out. One of the first things you may forget about when stressed is checking your blood sugar in the middle of the day. So for three whole days you hardly check at all, let alone before lunch. Now you've completely "screwed-up" that two-week period of checking before lunch each day according to your goal statement.

You can either: feel as if you've failed and decide to give up *or* give yourself the space to recover from the stressful life event or whatever threw you off-track and refocus when you are ready with the support of your Pick-Up Plan.

Your Pick-Up Plan:

1. **Acknowledging what happened:** *I'm really stressed-out and upset because my boyfriend broke up with me, work is stressful, and so I just don't have the energy to deal with my diabetes right now!*
2. **Supportive and positive self-talk:** *Okay, I'm just going through a lot right now—it's okay that I've fallen off-track for a moment. I'm human, and while I'd like to build the skills to keep diabetes on-track even during stressful times, that's not always possible, and that's okay. Take a deep breath.*
3. **Plan:** *I'm going to spend tomorrow relaxing (or at the gym or crying on the phone with a friend or watching reruns of Seinfeld all day) and just give myself space to calm down. The day after that, I'm going to refocus on my goal of checking my blood sugar before lunch for the next two weeks.*

Your Pick-Up Plan is about getting back on-track gradually without all of the guilt or negative nonsense of beating yourself up for simply falling off-track. Depending on the situation or the goal, each Pick-Up Plan can and probably will be different, but creating the habit, specifically in your head, of thinking through what happened and how you'll get back on track is what's most important.

When the Going Gets Tough …

As a personal trainer and a once competitive athlete myself, there was something I observed in both my clients and my own athletic challenges that I realized can make all the difference in reaching your goals. You see, there's a little secret that probably all people who have experienced success in some area of their life have learned: just because something is challenging doesn't make it a bad thing.

There's a certain point during a weightlifting workout, when the average person will feel her muscles start to burn and fatigue. I realized early on in my pursuit of competitive weightlifting that the moment I feel my muscles start to burn is when the real work begins. Yes, it's become challenging, even "painful" in a way that isn't actually detrimental pain, and our mind's natural instinct might be to say, "Okay, this is hard now. Let's stop."

But learning how to feel that burning muscle—or the challenge in any goal you're pursuing—and say to yourself, "Okay, giddy-up! Now it's time to really work!" is the key to making great strides in any goal you set out to accomplish.

During my first year as a personal trainer, I realized there were two kinds of clients: clients who feel that burn and give up unless I beg and beg and beg them to keep moving, and clients who feel that burn and say, "Oh, man, my muscles are burning!" and they *keep on going!*

Now, of course, in something like weightlifting, that point of difficulty can vary greatly from person to person depending on your age, your fitness, any injuries or health conditions, and that same logic can be applied to any goal, any challenge.

It's all about learning the difference between something that's truly negative and something that's truly just challenging. There will inevitably be moments in your goals around diabetes, nutrition, and exercise where you'll hit a point where it feels as if you cannot do what you set out to do. There will be moments when you'll think, "Ugh, this is so hard." Moments after that thought goes through your head, you can learn how to remind yourself that just because you're struggling doesn't mean you're doing poorly. Just because something has become seemingly impossible in any given moment (like choosing carrots and hummus over a bowl of ice cream) doesn't mean you're not doing well; it just means that in this moment, you have to work harder.

When I hit those moments in the gym, and I'd find myself struggling to move the weight in a specific exercise, I'd remind myself of my grandfather. He never stopped making improvements in himself. When he was 90 years old, he was studying new languages, trying to build his jogging strength up after knee replacement surgery, and always aiming to face his health challenges with perseverance.

When I found myself struggling in the gym and *wanting* to give up and put the weight down, I'd ask myself, "What would my grandfather expect from me in this moment?" Then I'd repeat over and over in my head, "*I can. I can. I can. I can. I can.*" While I repeated my mantra, I kept moving my body, pressing the weights, and working my way toward my athletic goals.

The simple sentence "I can" helped me overcome *many, many, many* moments of wanting to give up in many things. And, hey, it even helped me get back on the horse when I did give up momentarily on my goals!

And you can bet I had to do the same thing when it came to preparing for the weigh-ins before a meet, when I knew I had to eat very, very carefully in order to make it in the weight-class I wanted to compete in. When I suddenly got a craving for something more enticing and more delicious than chicken and vegetables, I had to remind myself of what I was after, why I was doing this. Those moments, albeit brief sometimes, were challenging, and had I given in to the cravings, I would've potentially sacrificed my athletic ambitions just because I let a challenging moment lead me to giving up.

And that's why I've taken the time to pinpoint phrases or statements that work well *for me, in my brain*, that I can reach for quickly and easily when I really need them. When the going gets tough …

These phrases can be corny, weird, confusing (to everyone besides you), really specific, or even really vague (yup, this is where you can finally be vague!).

Ginger's top five motivating statements:

1. I can. I can. I can. I can. I can. (*This one simply distracts me from the pain or challenge!*)
2. This is not supposed to be easy! (*A favorite saying of one of my first personal trainers, Norm.*)
3. I can always do just a little bit more. (*I think of my grandfather when I remind myself of this. I know I wouldn't want him to see me give up on anything!*)
4. Eye of the tiger. (*Yes, this one is corny, don't laugh! I love Rocky Balboa, and this phrase helps me focus on being tenacious and fearless!*)

5. I can accomplish anything I set my mind to. *(My brothers Dave and Pete are great examples of this mindset, and they inspire me to go after my goals and dreams completely!)*

Now, you guessed it, it's your turn.

Think of a few simple words, a simple phrase, a simple sentence that embodies what *you* need in order to remind yourself that those challenging moments are where the real work really happens.

Write down three to five different phrases or sentences:

_____

_____

_____

_____

_____

Now take a look at the list above and really think about what you're facing right now in your diabetes that you feel the most challenged by. Pick just one of those phrases to memorize, then write it down on sticky notes everywhere in your house and car and desk, smoosh that phrase into your brain so it's there when you really need to reach for it.

It Ain't So Easy!

Okay, so this chapter was all about creating awesome goals in relation to *anything*, but don't worry, I know it's not that simple. I'm sure you've heard this from an uninformed nondiabetic at least once in your life: "Oh, you have diabetes? You just have to, like, manage it, right? And you'll be fine?"

Um, yeah, except that whole "manage it" part is the really, really hard part.

In the next three chapters we're going to dig specifically into the three things that make diabetes complicated: blood sugars, food, and exercise.

What Others Have to Say

Riva Greenberg, living with type 1 diabetes
(DiabetesStories.com)

It's been 41 years since I was diagnosed and much has changed. When I was diagnosed there were no glucose meters available and I was put on one injection of insulin a day, in the morning.

Of course, the diagnosis was stressful. I was a freshman in college living away from home and I was put in the hospital for four days to regulate my blood sugar and learn how to inject insulin. I remember thinking my life was beginning and ending all at the same time. I also had a doctor in the hospital who had absolutely no bedside manner. He told me all the complications I was going to get and gave me two books to read about them. I was both distraught and yet at the same time it all felt dream-like.

Over the past three decades, as meters and more information have come out, I've learned how to take care of my diabetes and I'm grateful for every advance that makes it easier. Today, I take as many shots as I need, usually four to seven a day, and I'm not stressed at all by that. I'm grateful I can control my blood sugar so well. My daily management is pretty routine, which takes a lot of the stress out. I keep my meter in the same place in my apartment, test and eat around the same times, and eat the same type of foods for most meals.

I think it's the constant guessing and the frustration because you can't always guess correctly. Sometimes I think I should eat another few bites of something sweet because I think I need to raise my blood sugar a little. But then I'll discover it raises me too much. My body obviously has a mind of its own; it was doing something other than what I thought.

(continued)

(continued)

What Others Have to Say

Then there's the constant running in your head: When did I eat? What did I eat? Darn, I didn't plan on this walk when I took my insulin this morning! The constant tracking and adjustments that are just normal going through an ordinary day. People never understand how I can have diabetes 41 years and yet each day I have to figure it out all over again. And there's no sliding. You'd think you could just close your eyes to it one day, one weekend, but you can't without potential consequences.

I do get tired of diabetes. Then, when I just want a break, I don't check my blood sugar as much. I'll check a few times a day rather than six or seven. I'll usually skip the post-meal checks. I won't push myself to take my hour power walk and I will walk away from my computer, where it feels like all I do is spend time thinking and writing about diabetes, and I'll spend time with friends.

Ward Alper, living with type 2 diabetes
(TheDecadentDiabetic.com)

Because I took the management of my diabetes into my own hands by re-learning and re-inventing the way I cook and eat, my life in general has become less stressful. The most challenging thing about my life is meal planning. In the "old" days I was able to do pasta two nights a week and soup with bread two nights a week. I could boil up a batch of pasta and do something as easy as toss butter and cheese into it and dinner was done. Lunch used to be more stressful until I discovered Joseph's bread products. They have brought a normalcy back to my life. But dinner? Seven nights of planning even if I have leftover chicken … I still have to work at how to use it.

(continued)

(continued)

What Others Have to Say

For me, burnout happens when I am slapped in the face with a surprise situation. For example, I thought that a lunch of cottage cheese and fruit salad would be the perfect thing [for the diabetes diet]. That is until I started counting up the carbohydrates and discovered that what I thought of as fruit and cottage cheese was too high in carbohydrates. I knew how to make the adjustment but it just seemed to really bother me that what I always thought of as healthy "diet" food was not going to work. I just feel like I would like to scream. That stupid thing just seemed to overwhelm me.

But I have learned not to make too much of being a diabetic. It is not my nature to find things difficult. Sure, I miss some foods, but all in all it is not a big thing for me today.

My advice? Get over it. It is your disease, not your life. Kiss a lover, feed a bird. You are not to blame for being diabetic, it does not define you.

Brandy Barnes, living with type 1 diabetes
(DiabetesSisters.org)

My daughter, Summer, is my biggest motivating factor. I want her to see me as "strong and brave mommy," not "sick and weak mommy." I don't want any of her childhood memories to include—"Mommy was sick … she didn't feel good a lot." I also want to be here to help her through life's trials and tribulations, help her pick out her wedding dress, and help her pick out baby clothes one day. At the end of my life, I want to say, "I have lived a GOOD life!" and I don't want to have any regret like wishing I had taken better care of my diabetes. The only way to achieve that is to do all I can today and each and every day.

(continued)

(*continued*)

What Others Have to Say

Most importantly, I want to serve as a good role model for Summer. She watches everything I say and do. We have exercised together since she was very young—taking Zumba classes (yes, she was the youngest person in the class, but she held her own.), running together, and biking together. I grew up with parents who were very physically active and I know the positive impact it has had on me. I want to have that same impact on my daughter and pass on the tradition. We have had lots of conversations about what foods are healthy and what foods are not. Kids are known for telling it like it is, so she will let me know if she has seen me eating too many "unhealthy" foods. It's easy to get mad at your husband for saying, "Should you be eating that?" but when your daughter says, "Mommy, you've eaten a lot of chocolate this weekend," it's not nearly as maddening. It's more like a "wake-up call" than anything because I know her intent is truly genuine concern.

I heard someone say that having diabetes is like having another full-time job. There are days when I totally understand that statement because diabetes is taking so much of my time (and mental power) and there are days that I feel like that statement is giving diabetes too much power/control in my life. Diabetes is different every single day—which is a good thing and a bad thing!

Brian Cohen, living with type 2 diabetes
(TuDiabetes.org/profile/bsc)

When I was first diagnosed, the doctor gave me prescriptions for metformin and told me that all I had to do was take a pill and I would be "fine." Well, I'm not fine and I will never be fine. I have diabetes and it isn't just taking a pill and forgetting about it. It has seemingly invaded every part of my life and I have to think about it all the time, every day. Forever. And so, I will say it: diabetes is a mental problem. After my diagnosis back in 2005, I learned a lot

(*continued*)

(continued)

What Others Have to Say

about how to manage my diabetes. I would even consider myself an "expert" on the mechanics. But knowing how to do it and getting my head around doing it, that is the problem. So I know about how to take all my medications, count my carbs and dose my insulin. I know about the importance of exercise, I have the equipment and knowledge. For a while I was really fit, but I've had setbacks with my exercise and I know I need to get back on track, but mentally I just have not been able to get my head around it. I'm always tired, always have too little time. So I just got burned out with exercise and I continue to struggle to make the right decisions about exercise.

I have to do certain things to take care of myself and wherever possible I make these into rituals and things that are automatic. It isn't about making a decision, but about following a pattern. This has helped with a lot of things: taking medication, counting carbs, and dosing insulin. In other areas, I have had to turn to other approaches. Before my diagnosis, I had a terrible diet. After my diagnosis I struggled with the restrictions. I felt like it was always about what I couldn't eat.

What really helped was to turn things around to identify what I liked and enjoyed. And amazingly, the glass is half-full and there is a huge world of things I can eat that are still a big part of my enjoyment in life. I think the same thing can be said about exercise—it is a matter of finding things you like.

The easiest part of managing diabetes has turned out to be diet. And I don't mean easy in terms of level of difficulty or time, I mean easiest as an element of my life that I am happy about. I have become a really good cook. I purchase really good ingredients and really enjoy food. Yes, I spend an hour or so every day in the kitchen and some hours every week scouring the stores, but it has become something I enjoy and want to do. That makes it easy.

(continued)

(continued)

What Others Have to Say

Scott Strange, living with type 1 diabetes
(StrangelyDiabetic.com)

My management goes on "autopilot" when I'm burned-out. I still test and count carbs, but I get very reactive to things instead of trying to be more proactive. Diabetes is so ingrained in my day-to-day life that any type of burnout I am experiencing also flips that "autopilot" switch to ON.

To get through a burnout, some of the stress has to be eliminated. Either through talking it out with my support network or my getting away from it somehow (with a vacation, movie, etc.).

I believe that burnout is perfectly normal and to be expected from time to time. Folks may be uncomfortable admitting it (especially men), but I believe that we will all experience it. We may deal with it privately or more openly, but however it is dealt with, the important thing is that it works for you.

I also believe that it is okay to ask for help. Diabetes may be one of the most demanding patient-managed conditions on the planet. No matter what type you have, it sucks, and it is an immense help to have support. Asking for that help, whatever the type, may be one of the hardest, yet most rewarding things you can do for yourself.

Self-care is critical for people with chronic conditions. I'm not talking about the mechanics of dosing insulin and counting carbs, I mean emotional self-care. There will be good days, bad days, and days where you just don't give a damn. Find some support, especially peer support from folks who are going through exactly what you are. We're not just a diagnosis, we're complete beings whose emotional and mental needs are just as important as the physical ones. Don't forget that, and know you are not alone in this.

(continued)

(continued)

What Others Have to Say

Bob Pederson, living with type 2 diabetes
(Tminustwo.net)

After an early childhood of being chronically underweight, something changed during the fourth grade: I was chubby by the end of that year and seriously overweight by my mid-teens. By age 48, I'd been 100-plus pounds overweight for 25 years or more. I had never thought this was a good idea and had made various efforts to lose weight over the years.

When I was diagnosed [with type 2 diabetes], I hoped that the seriousness of my situation would enable me to make big changes. My failure to make those changes brought what I think I can call burnout almost right away. It was not until I abandoned significant weight loss as a goal in favor of focusing on how I live that I started making such progress as I have made.

Though it took me several years to really figure it out, and I grouse ceaselessly about filling my pill sorters, I've really gotten pretty good at staying on top of the dozen or so prescriptions and supplements I take at three separate times of day.

Because I am a lifelong depressive, my physical health and mental health are in a constant elaborate dance. In the best times, self-care comes easily. In the worst times, there are no resources available for anything beyond getting through my days. Burnout and discouragement about self-care are a part of that dance. When the level of discouragement and burnout is strong, I tend to pretty much abandon my efforts to be better.

But I've learned over the years that discouragement lies. It will tell you that things are worse than they are, that you are less than you are, and that your unhappiness will last forever. It's like looking in a funhouse mirror: we have to remember that our perceptions are not always reliable. Also, in my experience anyway, it is unwise to plan changes when discouragement is strong.

(continued)

(*continued*)

What Others Have to Say

Asha Brown, living with type 1 diabetes
(WeAreDiabetes.org)

The first years of living with diabetes were emotionally unmemorable for me. My dad has type 1 diabetes, and when my parents found out that I also had it, I was simply sent home after the diagnosis appointment with insulin, syringes, and an apologetic pat on the head. My parents took excellent care of me, and when I reached the age that I wanted to have sleepovers with my best friend, they told me that in order for me to do that I had to learn how to be more proactive about my diabetes. I think I was giving myself my own injections by age 7.

Until the seventh grade. In seventh grade I was bullied by some of my teachers. Although my parents did an excellent job of providing information to all my teachers about type 1 diabetes, a number of my seventh grade teachers did not seem to understand that people living with diabetes will sometimes miss school and can get sick more easily, etc.

They asked me if they could expect to see better attendance (I had been very sick with mono for a few weeks and my blood sugars had been all over the place so I had missed a few days of school) and they wanted to see "improvement in my diabetes" in the future. I was so confused. Did they mean that I was a bad diabetic? Was it because I tested my blood sugar during school too much? Were there other type 1 diabetics my age who had better numbers than me who never missed school? I was so embarrassed and simply nodded my head and left that room with so much shame. I didn't even know why I felt ashamed. I only knew one thing; my diabetes made me weak. After that experience, a lot changed emotionally for me.

(*continued*)

(continued)

What Others Have to Say

I spent 10 years of my life knowing I wasn't doing the right thing; living in denial of my diabetes and trying to *will* my diabetes into the shadows of my life instead of allowing it to be a very large part of who I truly am. On a day where I take my insulin to cover a meal only to find that I am sky high or really low a few hours after the meal, I deal with it and try to avoid playing any head games with myself about it.

If I allow myself to "play the victim" for what I have to go through on a daily basis in order to stay alive and stay healthy, I have to live with that anger, fear, and anxiety. I find that acceptance and action—even when I'm angry at the pharmacy for messing up my lantus order for the hundredth time and when I'm exhausted and don't want to pull myself out of bed to test before I go to sleep—are much better choices than allowing the burned-out feeling to "win."

Diabetes burnout comes in an emotional form for me. I have a few days every year where I can literally blame every single bad thing that has happened to me on my diabetes ... student loans for a degree that is unfinished because I was battling diabulimia through college ... responding to my body's aches and pains (frozen shoulder, nerve damage, polycystic ovary syndrome, and an altogether extremely fragile immune system) with deep remorse and sadness for the years I spent punishing my body instead of trying to help it.

Feeling burned-out with a chronic illness can and does pass, but neglecting my health results in permanent damage and I want to live as full and pain-free of a life as I can for as long as possible!

(continued)

(*continued*)

What Others Have to Say

Beatriz Dominguez, living with type 2 diabetes
(CrankyPancreas.com)

Type 2 diabetes is tricky. Everything is about what you eat, what you do, being disciplined when taking medication. I don't use insulin, and many times I'm frustrated by the fact that there is no way for me to control what carbohydrates do to my blood glucose levels if I'm not careful. And most of the time I feel like it's a lottery; sometimes I eat something horrible and my glucose metabolism doesn't even blink, while other times I wonder what my cells are thinking when what I put in my mouth couldn't be healthier. I love to eat, and I love to eat the kind of food that tastes so good you know it's going to be bad. I have to be honest and admit that more often than not I play blood sugar roulette and pay for it later.

I really don't think there is an easy aspect of diabetes management, but the one I have the least issues with is keeping my doctor's appointments regular no matter what's going on in my life. There are times when I don't feel like going because I know numbers and such will be bad, but I remind myself that it's better to be there. I do follow-up appointments, see specialists I'm referred to, and try to be organized with my calendars when it comes to medical care; it's a priority.

I honestly forget that I have a glucose meter. Having type 2 diabetes makes it worse, especially because I don't use insulin so I don't have to test often. That and the fact that I was told to test as needed. So there are times when I fall off the wagon and I don't test for days … or weeks. Mostly because I get discouraged by the fact that diabetes is such a roller coaster, but also because at some point we all want to pretend diabetes doesn't exist.

(*continued*)

(*continued*)

What Others Have to Say

I just keep reminding myself that I have to do better. I learned not to be so hard on myself just recently. Nobody's perfect, and diabetes doesn't take breaks from us and we should try our best to keep up with it.

Cynthia Zuber, living with type 1 diabetes
(DiabetesLight.com)

For most of the 26 years I have lived with type 1 diabetes, I don't think I ever experienced "classic burnout." I have always been one of those diligent patients who test their blood sugar 7 to 10 times every day and faithfully takes her insulin, eats a pretty healthy diet (while still allowing for treats, of course!), exercises (at least occasionally, for the first many years), etc. Surprising even to myself, the last one to two years of my life living with diabetes have been the most challenging— I have experienced the most tears, the most frustration, the most flat-out disappointment in the effects diabetes has had on my life.

But, the truth? I see this as a sign of health! You see, for soooo many years (most of my life, really), I just accepted it all! No questions asked. I dealt with things and moved on. What I really became an expert on was not even allowing myself to feel the feelings diabetes was causing and just push them under the rug. Now, I will cry my eyes out. I might talk to my husband, some good friends with diabetes, or my blog's Facebook community.

I believe excellent self-care involves tending not only to our physical health but to our emotional health as well. If I am feeling angry, sad, or frustrated, I go for a walk or a bike ride. Exercising brings a sense of clarity and positiveness that I really can do this another day. More importantly, it restores balance to my thoughts,

(*continued*)

(continued)

What Others Have to Say

allowing me to feel and release negative emotions. This, in turn, allows me to see the myriad blessings all around me and smile despite the hardships this life with diabetes presents.

As I've matured, I've learned to give myself patience and love when I fall off-track from ways of caring for myself that are not in my best self-interest. I have sought the help of a trusted therapist to work through areas needing growth. By learning to love myself in places that need nurturing and talking through my struggles with someone educated to help create positive change, I have worked through many of the barriers that used to hold me back! This has led to vast improvement in my physical, mental, and emotional health. Now when I am feeling stuck, I remember how much more successful I am when I extend love and acceptance toward myself rather than shame and criticism.

When Every Little Number Feels Like a Grade

4

Taking on the Responsibilities of Medications and Blood Sugar Checks without the Overwhelming Pressure

This morning, I woke up with a blood sugar of 246 mg/dL. And believe me, seeing this number was more than simply disappointing, it was also momentarily *infuriating* because I went to bed with a blood sugar of 120 mg/dL and all the insulin I needed for a fairly low-carb dinner of pork, bell peppers, and a half-cup of black beans.

Two things went through my mind after seeing that number, and these are two things that often go through my mind on the days when I have a high blood sugar in the morning:

1. Ugh, that means I was probably high for most of the night, which means over time that will impact my next A1C test. And, in general, that's another seven hours of my life that was spent with a high blood sugar, and seven hours of my life that will increase the risk of losing my vision, fingers, toes, and kidneys. Grr!

2. Ugh, that means that if I actually let my doctor print out the numbers from my meter at my next appointment, she's going to see that 246 mg/dL and circle it with her red marker and say, "Oh my, so what happened here?" as if every high blood sugar has a memorable explanation, even if it happened two months before my appointment.

And that's when I realized why I woke up with such a high number. I had used the very last bits of my bottle of Lantus insulin but the insulin had expired—even though it had not been a full month since opening it. (I swear! I checked!)

Allow me to explain, that just like many others with type 1 or type 2 diabetes, I have high blood sugars now and then throughout any week, but they really only drive me nuts when I can't determine what caused the high, especially when I feel as if I did everything I was supposed to do. I *don't* get frustrated by highs after eating moderate-to-high carbohydrate meals that are difficult to measure and difficult to estimate the carbohydrates in, because I know that I was in a situation with several variables that weren't so easy to balance considering my body isn't capable of producing insulin. In those situations, I actually check my blood sugar one to two hours after a meal just to see if I can catch the potential high and correct it sooner than later.

But this high blood sugar, this darn 246 mg/dL wasn't my fault, you see. Still, I know that no matter how I explain it to my doctor at my next appointment, she's going to lecture me about it.

"Well," she'll say, "You should mark your vials after you open them."

"Um," I'll say, "but it's definitely been less than 30 days since I opened this, and I'm usually in the mindset of '*Must not waste insulin. Use the last drop. This disease is so expensive!*'"

She'll probably let it go after that, but the very light lecture and the furrowed brow will have already happened. And the memory of her furrowed brow will crawl onto my shoulders and sit there, with all the other furrowed brows or lectures that have come from magazines, strangers, doctors, parents, TV, and friends. And it will just add to that daily pressure of feeling like I should be the perfect diabetic even though, to anyone who is paying attention, it obviously isn't possible or realistic.

Have you ever been part of a conversation that was some version of this:

Concerned Person: You need to start taking better care of your diabetes.
Person with Diabetes: Um, yes, I know. I know.
Concerned Person: If you don't get your A1C down, you could end up losing your feet, your fingers, your vision, and your kidneys.
Person with Diabetes: Um, yes …
Concerned Person: Be scared. Be very scared.

I don't know about you, but fear doesn't really motivate me; neither do threats or diabetes horror stories. Motivation comes from many places, but for most people it doesn't come from fear. And yet, from the day we are diagnosed, everyone tries to motivate us through fear, scary stories about losing our feet, and threats to take away things that make us happy if we don't become perfectly "compliant" in life with diabetes.

"Compliant." Geez. What a great word. Yuck.

Being "compliant" doesn't inspire me. What inspires me, personally, is thinking about the things I want in my future. The things I want to experience, accomplish, and be alive for. There is a major difference between being afraid of losing your eyesight to retinopathy due to high blood sugars and being *motivated* by the idea of having wonderful, amazing eyesight when I'm older despite my diabetes!

One approach about fueling fear. It feels threatening. Scary. Unfair. And cruel.

And the other choice looks forward at what you or I want for our lives, for our future. I *want* to have sparkling, healthy eyes and awesome fingers and toes when I'm older … and so, I check my blood sugar regularly and try to maintain a healthy A1C level. I'm not focusing on avoiding retinopathy and going blind and scary images of people who've endured leg amputations, I'm focusing—every day—on the continued goal of being *healthy and happy* as I grow older.

I am inspired on a daily basis to manage my diabetes because I want to grow old with my soon-to-be husband, Roger. Because I love jumping around in the gym, lifting things, pushing things, pulling things. Because I want to write more books. Because I love running around in the snow with my dogs and getting dragged down our dirt road during daily walks by all three of them on leashes. I am inspired on a daily basis because I want to have a baby, create a family, and be healthy enough to take care of that family for many years to come. I want to meet my best friend Tara for dinner and movies when we're old and gray. I want to teach yoga to senior citizens when I'm 70 years old. I want to be a grandmother who is healthy and active and *alive* for as long as possible.

I am inspired on a daily basis to manage my diabetes, partly because someday there might be a cure for diabetes, and I want to be healthy enough to receive that cure, but also because I want my future, or even simply tomorrow, to be full of possibilities.

And you know, in the end, I just like *feeling good*. Feeling energetic. Feeling happy. As soon as diabetes management goes out the window, those three things, I know, go with it. But believe me, that doesn't mean I'm all "Yay! Let's manage diabetes today!" all the time. I'm sick of dealing with diabetes every day. *Every* day. But I keep checking my blood sugar, taking my insulin, and counting my carbohydrates because it keeps my life full of possibilities.

What do you want in your future? Tomorrow, next year, or 10 years from now?

No matter what it is, our life with diabetes today matters, but the most we can *all* do is giving our best one day at a time.

It Takes Two to Tango at the Doctor's Office

Chances are if you've gone to a restaurant at least five times in your life, you've experienced the array of quality one can find in a waiter or waitress. (I believe the politically correct term these days is "server.") Some are wonderful: they smile, chat with you just enough to be friendly but not so long that they stop doing their job, and they actually bring you what you ordered.

Others, not so much: they mumble, barely look you in the eyes if at all, and they bring you regular Coke instead of Diet because they figured it hardly mattered anyway … or they forget you actually ordered a Diet—either reason isn't good.

Just like the staff in any restaurant, or the teachers in your high school, some health care professionals are great and some are not so great. And that's why you can't settle for a doctor who isn't providing the care and support you need in your life with diabetes.

Believe me, I've met my share of rude, arrogant, lousy doctors and nurses, but fortunately, there are also a tremendous amount of great, awesome, thoughtful, compassionate doctors and nurses and diabetes educators out there, too.

But it takes two to tango. (Yes, the title of this section wasn't random!)

We need doctors (or nurse practitioners or certified diabetes educators (CDEs)) who are able to treat us like human beings rather than just patients with diabetes. They'll listen to our concerns, our questions, our fears. They'll look us in the eye and speak thoughtfully when addressing the fact that maybe we need to lose weight or maybe our A1C has increased significantly since our last appointment. They won't scold or blame or boo and hiss at our imperfections. And they won't let us settle for less than our best—they'll challenge us, motivate us, encourage us to keep trying.

But we need to *show up*, too, and I don't just mean, like, check in at the front desk and sit down in the doctor's office. I mean totally show up, 100 percent. There is no health care professional in the world who can help us if we ourselves don't listen, ask questions, tell the truth—make an effort.

In my experience as a diabetes coach, sometimes the biggest source of diabetes burnout is just frustration with blood sugars that don't seem to budge despite your best efforts … and quite often the solution is a few simple tweaks in your insulin doses! But if you don't explain what's going on to your doctor, and don't let him *help you* with your insulin doses, then diabetes will continue to be that much harder.

Sometimes, what needs the most attention is merely how you communicate with your doctor or CDE. Strengthening this aspect of your relationship, so that each appointment can make a world of difference!

Here are a few tips for you, as the patient, and then, a few tips for your doctor or CDE. (If you can't bare the idea of *telling* your doctor or CDE how to improve their communication during your appointment, make a copy of this page and mail it to them anonymously!)

Three Things to Remember When Visiting Your Doctor

1. Try Asking the Question, "If I Could Focus on Improving One Habit in My Life, Which Part of My Life Would You Suggest I Focus On: Exercise, Nutrition, or Diabetes Management?"

Sometimes, especially if you've been struggling with your health and diabetes overall, your doctor may give you a very vague form of advice simply because she doesn't have enough time to break apart every aspect of your health that needs to be improved upon. And, naturally, your doctor may realize that telling you to make improvements in all three areas could simply be overwhelming. Show your doctor that you're interested by asking for the suggestions yourself, and give her permission to help you focus on just one area rather than all three.

2. Stand Up for Yourself

If it feels as if your doctor has suddenly forgotten just how challenging diabetes is, speak up. Remind her that balancing your blood sugar around *life* isn't easy. That knowing the carbohydrates in everything you eat *all the time* isn't really possible. That you get *zero* days off from the demands of diabetes. That you're doing the best you can. Some doctors may be so overwhelmed by a day full of patients, all of whom may have diabetes, that you may be getting mixed up in the mash of people they are trying to help attain better blood sugars. And I'm not excusing them, but … *stand up for yourself* if you feel that your own doctor is not treating you like an individual.

3. Always Ask More Questions

These days, health care professionals of all kinds are under a major time-crunch, so if you don't stop and ask them for more details, more information, they may just graze right by you. (Of course, it couldn't hurt to write your questions down on paper and keep that piece of paper in your hand to ensure your questions come up during your appointment.) At the start of each appointment, a nurse probably checks your blood pressure and your weight. If the nurse doesn't volunteer the information—and they usually don't—ask what those numbers are! (You could even ask to have all the numbers written down so you can take them home with you—it's easy to forget all those test results by the time you're back to your busy life.) If your doctor makes changes in your insulin doses or your oral medications that you don't understand, *ask* why she made those changes. The more effort you put into learning about your diabetes and your health during those appointments, the more you'll get out of them.

Three Questions Every Doctor Should Ask You

The following three questions are something you should consider printing out and handing to your doctor. Sometimes, the most important questions our doctors could ask us are the most basic, and yet, with a day full of patients to see, these questions can be the first thing your doctor doesn't make time for.

If you're not too fond of your current doctor and overall health care team, and they don't seem to be listening to *you* the individual, or asking you at least *one* of these questions during your appointments, it may be time to start finding a new doctor!

1. What Have Been Some of the Biggest Challenges for You concerning Your Health Lately?

This question is purposefully open-ended. Doctors might look at our blood sugars and think they can pinpoint exactly what's wrong, but the numbers are only half the story. It may look as if I need more basal insulin during the night because I'm waking up with high blood sugars when what's really causing the highs may be binge-eating before bed because I'm going through a divorce or struggling with depression or really stressed-out at work. Whatever it is, the number doesn't tell the whole story. Asking this open-ended question gives the patient room to say exactly what's been the hardest, and that will often directly explain why blood sugars may be out of whack during a particular part of the day.

2. How Can I Help You Today?

This open-ended question addresses the same issue of assuming what we, the patient, need rather than letting us tell the doctor. Using the same example of high blood sugars in the morning, I may know exactly why they're high (because of overeating late at night or forgetting to take my insulin, etc.), but what I really want to talk to my doctor about might be something completely different, which is possibly much more important!

3. Do You *Know You're Doing a* Really Great *Job?*

This question should be asked of *everybody* … even the patients whose blood sugars may not look so stellar. Too often, we feel judged and guilty when we're with our doctor. The focus is always on what we *aren't* doing well, which numbers *aren't* in range, how we're *not* exercising enough or we gained *too much* weight, etc. But before all those details is this disease. And this disease is *hard, hard, hard work!* To hear from our doctors that they understand we're doing the best we can (even when our best doesn't look all that great) and that they understand how immensely challenging diabetes and health care can be, can easily change how open and eager we as patients are to opening up and talking to our doctors. It doesn't matter what our A1C is, or if we've been diagnosed with type 1 or type 2 or type 1.5 diabetes, we deserve a pat on the back just for showing up every day.

Step Away from the Number

Unfortunately, in a sense, each number on our meter is sort of a grade, right? I mean, we can sugarcoat this, but the truth is that each number is a reflection of our ability to handle the crazy demands of this crazy disease. Just because it's impossible to do it perfectly doesn't take away from the fact that we feel as if we ought to be doing it perfectly, and it doesn't change how it feels to see a 235 mg/dL on our glucose meter when we were hoping to see something more like 104 mg/dL. While this book isn't really about *how* to attain better blood sugars, there is a simple fact that remains: there is always more to learn about blood sugar and diabetes management. Always. Not only is there literally more information to learn about the variety of physiological variables that change how our bodies use glucose, produce hormones that raise glucose or increase insulin resistance, etc. etc. etc., there's also simply our own ability to problem solve and learn about our own diabetes.

If I'm constantly high after eating breakfast, but I don't take the time to stop and figure out how much insulin I actually need at breakfast or how to alter what I'm eating so it doesn't have as much of an impact on my blood sugar, then I'm skipping a really useful aspect of how I see each number on my meter.

It's information. It's telling me how the food I just ate affected my blood sugar. It's telling me how accurate my insulin dose or oral medication doses are. It's telling me whether the kind of exercise I just did burned more glucose or more body fat. It's all information.

We can see the information and get pissed off and depressed. Or we can use it to keep tweaking, keep learning, and keep trying.

In my own life, my insulin needs have changed drastically during the past year due to weight-loss and major changes in how I eat and exercise. And while the fluctuating numbers have been frustrating (particularly the 3:00 a.m. blood sugars around 40 mg/dL), I have reminded myself constantly that they are information reflecting the many changes going on in my life that have had major impacts on my body's insulin needs.

The other option would be to see these crazy blood sugar fluctuations and say, "Diabetes is so crazy! It doesn't make sense! Nothing ever works! I can't do this!" But that wouldn't get me anywhere.

Instead, I have spent several *months* constantly adjusting my doses bit-by-bit, as my weight has continued to drop and my sensitivity to insulin has continued to increase. Bit-by-bit. Creating "experiments" around my doses to see if they are accurate, and taking good notes. Bit-by-bit.

Diabetes isn't easy, but it isn't random either. Every number holds information. Changing the way you see those numbers will change the way you respond to them, which will change the way you manage your diabetes, and one day, you'll find yourself learning through those numbers, rather than judging yourself.

Like I Said, My Fingers Hurt!

But … that doesn't mean pricking your finger day in and day out isn't totally obnoxious. So obnoxious that, hey, maybe you don't want to check your blood sugar very often anymore like you're "supposed to"? Swallowing all those pills? And the injections? The pumps, pods, and continuous glucose monitors? You're sick of it? You forget to do it? Forget you have diabetes? Hey, look, you're not alone, and I wish I could truly forget I have diabetes, too. Diabetes sucks!

The biggest glitch in the whole, "You need to check your blood sugar at least four times a day" doctor's order is that even though, combined, this task takes up less than 120 seconds of our day, it's a tedious responsibility that comes with "good" or "bad" news depending on whatever our blood sugar is. If you're sick of diabetes and struggling with your numbers overall, then who could blame you for *not* wanting to stop in the middle of your day and get a reminder that you're not a perfect diabetic?

What if, instead of feeling as if you're a total failure for *not* checking your blood sugar at least four times a day like your doctor, mom, dad, husband, boyfriend, girlfriend, uncle—whoever—has ordered you to … what if you make a conscious choice to back off a bit? Instead of backing off totally and checking barely once a day or purposefully rebelling due to being sick of it all, what if you decide, "Okay, I need to lighten up on all this pressure. I'm going to focus on testing two to three times a day. And that's okay."

Yes, I understand that your mom might gasp at the idea of purpose-fully checking your blood sugar only twice a day, but if intentionally backing off on the pressure helps you recharge that overloaded diabetes management battery, then it's really okay!

Think about the current pressure that you (or someone else) have put on yourself regarding checking your blood sugar, and why it might feel like it is *too much* or *too stressful*. What is it, literally, in your own words and mind, about checking your blood sugar that causes you to avoid or forget to do it? Whatever the reason is, it matters. It's valid. It's important. But you've gotta get it out into words in order to move through it.

*In my head, I expect myself to check my blood sugar*_____
times a day, but this feels stressful or overwhelming because _____
_____.

In my work as a coach and mentor, I've asked many people to fill in those blanks, and sometimes it might take a while to express exactly what's going on in your head. Sometimes, the answer is as simple as, *I'm really &%$#ing angry I have diabetes.* Sometimes it might be, *Everybody keeps nagging me to check my blood sugar, so I fight back by not checking at all.* Or maybe it's about seeing the number on the screen and the pressure of having to figure out what to do about that number all the time.

Then create a purposeful, thoughtful plan to back-off on that pressure using what you've learned about creating awesome goal statements to focus on this aspect of your life with diabetes. (We'll talk in Chapter 7 about communicating this to your loved ones.) But remember, start slow! Here are a few examples of goal statements that ease into blood sugar checking:

- *I will check my blood sugar once a day, in the morning, for two weeks.*
- *I will check my blood sugar before breakfast and dinner, each day, for two weeks.*
- *I will aim to check my blood sugar a total of 10 times a week for two weeks.*

You might be looking at the above statements and thinking, "That's way less than what I'm really supposed to do," but if expecting 100 percent perfection leads you to checking your blood sugar almost never, then backing way off and creating an expectation that you can meet successfully will help you get back in the groove of checking more often down the road.

Here are a few tips to help you make checking your blood sugar a more regular part of your day:

- **Pick one part of the day that is *really* consistent in your life**—like brushing your teeth before bed—and create a mental habit of always checking your blood sugar whenever you brush your teeth before bed. For me, I take my dogs for a walk in the woods every morning, so the first thing I do *before* that walk is check my fasting blood sugar.

- **Keep your meter in the same place whenever you're at home or at work.** For instance, create a space on your desk (yes, right on top) where your meter will live when you're at work. At home, pick a space on the kitchen counter or the coffee table where your meter will always live. This way, it's in a visible area that you'll pass by many times a day.
- **Use all that technology!** I'm sure 75 percent of the people reading this book are obsessed with their smartphones … so use your smartphone to help you! The *best* diabetes app by far is "mySugr" but there are many others! Or at the very least, schedule your phone to alert you at a certain time of day to check your blood sugar.
- **Ask for help.** See if someone you live with, or someone you see almost every day, would be willing to ask you once a day, "Have you checked your blood sugar recently?" If that phrase sounds annoying, think of a clever way that they could remind you about checking your blood sugar that would actually feel supportive.
- **Think of your meter like it's your newborn baby.** If you have a tendency to leave the house without your meter, it might as well be like leaving your newborn baby at home! You need that meter in order to ensure your safety, so making it a priority to at least bring it with you everywhere—even if you don't use it every time you're out and about—can help develop your overall awareness of checking your blood sugar more often.

Even though blood sugar checking literally takes 120 seconds of the day, it is a big deal in many ways, and you have every right to hate doing it, to wish you didn't have to, and to want to forget about it altogether! But the reality is that it's a part of our lives.

Anxiety and Low Blood Sugars

The worst low blood sugar I've ever experienced was early in my powerlifting days. I'd just come home from a grueling training session, to my tiny studio apartment where my bedroom and kitchen were basically the same room, and had sat down on the floor in front of my bed (also known as my "couch") to watch television while I ate dinner. What I'd forgotten to do, though, was cut back on my insulin dose for dinner because I had just finished a very intense training session! Instead of taking three units of fast-acting insulin, I took six units. At that time in my life, one unit of insulin could lower my blood sugar about 75 points, so you can imagine the trouble I was in for when you consider that my blood sugar was around 140 mg/dL before I ate dinner.

Within about 30 minutes, I started fading and realized quickly the mistake I had made.

My hands were suddenly shaking, I was sweaty and hot, my vision was "screwy," and I felt like I couldn't speak. Crawling, I made my way from the floor next to my bed over to the kitchen counter (fortunately, like I said, my apartment was tiny so this was only about a six-foot crawl). On the edge of the counter was a large container of oatmeal, and it's all I could do to reach up and grab it, pouring some raw oatmeal down my throat. (Certainly not the world's most quickly digested carbohydrate, and who knows how in the world I was able to chew it without choking on it!)

While it probably would've been best to stay right there and wait patiently (or, um, gain the strength to get a juice box from the cabinet), I remember crawling back over to the bed and texting my trainer, Andrew, who was really the only person in my life at the time who lived in the area and knew much about diabetes.

I sent him a very mangled text explaining that I was having a really bad low blood sugar.

And then I passed out, face-first, in the carpet. I woke up about 30 minutes later to the sound of my phone—a text message from Andrew—asking if I was okay. (To his credit, I'm sure he was a little confused, since I hadn't typed very clearly and I'd never had a severe low before, so he had no idea just how bad of a deal I was in).

But I was okay, and it was scary.

To this day, I've never had a low blood sugar that left me unable to give myself food, but I owe part of that to the fact that I am truly afraid of ever being in that situation, so I am constantly on the lookout for the earlier symptoms of a low blood sugar.

For me, the first things I generally feel are heat (as in, my whole body just feels warmer) and an inability to concentrate. I've trained myself to get better and better at recognizing and responding to the most subtle versions of these symptoms. The moment I sense a feeling of being low, I can't get it out of my mind: I have to go check my blood sugar. Sometimes, especially in the middle of the night, the other part of my brain will say, "C'mon, I'm tired, go back to bed," but that part of me that is terrified of having a seizure keeps insisting, "No way. Get up. Go check."

Fear, in this situation, keeps me safe.

While high blood sugars may be more detrimental to our health in the long term, *low blood sugars* have a much great fear-factor. It's always amusing to hear a nondiabetic say, "I think my blood sugar is low" simply because they've gone too long without eating a meal. Sure, for a nondiabetic a blood sugar of 70 mg/dL would feel low, but for anyone with diabetes who takes insulin you know that there's a big difference between true hypoglycemia and having gone too long between breakfast and lunch.

Low blood sugars, generally anything below 70 mg/dL, can vary tremendously in their severity of symptoms. Some lows come on quickly because there's simply too much insulin and not enough glucose on board—something we've all experienced due to having to constantly estimate carbohydrate counts and insulin doses or balance our blood sugars during exercise. (To learn more about balancing your blood sugar when eating or exercising, check out my first book, *Your Diabetes Science Experiment*.) And of course, there's the slow and steady lows that can come on from busy activity such as shopping and vacuuming the house, and of course: going too long between meals!

Regardless of the cause, low blood sugars can be scary. So scary, in fact, that you may have gotten into the habit of purposefully leaving your blood sugars higher to prevent ever being low again! And hey, I don't blame you, because some low blood sugars can feel like we are dying. Like our brain is slowly shutting down. Our limbs. Our eyes. Our lips. Our ability to even communicate real language or a basic sentence. Seizures. They can be life-threatening. That's a fact.

Low blood sugars are scary. You have every right to feel anxious and nervous and extremely annoyed that you have to prevent these kinds of low blood sugars every single day. Fact!

But, if you're at a point in your life where you want to work your way back to feeling okay with an in-range blood sugar (let's say, under 160 mg/dL) rather than running in the high 200s and 300s all day, you'll have to start gradually. Part of the process of overcoming that anxiety is about rebuilding your confidence in your ability to maintain healthier blood sugars more often *and* in your ability to simply *treat* and *survive* low blood sugars!

Overall, there are a few careful steps you can take to help yourself work back toward healthier blood sugars while reducing your stress around going low:

1. **Create a new "range" to aim for.** If your body has been enduring very high blood sugars for many weeks or months, then your body has also literally adjusted to having a higher than normal glucose. This means that suddenly being at 120 mg/dL could actually feel very low and be very stressful. Instead of going from really high blood sugars to aiming for perfect blood sugars, talk to your doctor about actually aiming for blood sugars around 180 to 250 mg/dL. Over time, maybe after a month or two, you can start to aim for 160 mg/dL.

    Either way, be very specific. Make a conscious decision about what you will make your new "target range," and write it down on a big piece of paper that you'll stick to your refrigerator or bathroom mirror. That is your new normal.

2. **Create an experiment to build your confidence.** If you've been taking your insulin doses without measuring, and therefore you're truly unsure of just how many units of insulin you need for how many grams of carbohydrates, it's time to sit down with your health care team and fine-tune your insulin doses so they're accurate. If you can't trust that the insulin you're taking is indeed how much insulin you need, then no wonder you're terrified of going low! For example, if my blood sugar is 200 mg/dL and I want it to *stay* at 200 mg/dL because I'm working to avoid going too low, I would count my carbohydrates, take a specific amount of insulin, and check my blood sugar again at one hour and two hours to see how well the dose kept me at 200 mg/dL. This is the very simplified version of an "insulin-to-carbohydrate ratio experiment" and you can learn more about how to do this in my book *Your Diabetes Science Experiment.*

    And while you're at it, speaking of confidence, feel free to surround yourself with juice boxes and glucose tabs in every nook and cranny. Being prepared is half the battle when it comes to treating low blood sugars.

3. **Lighten up on the pressure.** Yes, we've all been told a thousand times that our blood sugars ought to be between 80 and 120 mg/dL all damn day, but that kind of pressure isn't what you need if you're struggling with anxiety around lows that are causing you to keep your blood sugars high. Instead, focus on what you truly need emotionally. Remind yourself that you're dealing with something major and you need time to readjust your blood sugars.

   This is about the message you're telling yourself. The mantra, so to speak. If while you're trying to overcome your anxiety around lows, you're also scolding yourself for having a high blood sugar, it won't be surprising if you're feeling a little under-motivated, eh? Think about the message you need to hear when you're in the midst of making a decision about your insulin dosing and your blood sugar. A kind message. A message that supports both you and your goal.

   It's a process! Take your time and be good to yourself.

The Blood Sugar Roller Coaster (Is So Annoying!)

This one is also for people taking insulin, because while those *not* taking insulin can experience highs and lows, they usually don't swing high or low very quickly and then swing in the other direction, unless you're on insulin. The crazy balance (or imbalance) between insulin and carbohydrates and hormones and exercise are the catalysts for that roller coaster.

Actually I'm taking a risk here with this one because my beliefs about roller coasters in life with diabetes may not be a popular one. I can't tell you how often I hear stories about random blood sugars, crazy mysterious highs, and inexplicable lows. Hey, I was convinced that's what I was once experiencing, too … until I stopped making excuses and decided to own every decision I made about my diabetes.

If I decide to snack all afternoon on random foods or eat a really delicious and sugary dessert, then I'm basically setting myself up for a possible high or even low blood sugar, especially if I just take a big dollop of insulin rather than trying to calculate an accurate dose, right? And that doesn't mean

I shouldn't necessarily enjoy the dessert, but I shouldn't be surprised if I end up with screwy blood sugars for the next several hours. In fact, personally, I anticipate those screwy blood sugars and try to preempt them by checking my blood sugar several times in the two hours following that mysterious dessert!

But the point is that aside from the moments when we're truly dealing with adrenaline rushes during competitive events or other physiological processes that are out of our control, there *are* many things we do ourselves that lead to that roller coaster. That doesn't mean we necessarily need to feel guilty about that, but it certainly isn't worth being surprised and frustrated if we *know* that the way we are behaving around food isn't exactly conducive to diabetes management.

Of course, even when we do find ourselves on the roller coaster, regardless of how we got there, there are other things we can do to help ensure we don't make the ride longer than it has to be.

Three Tips for Getting off the Blood Sugar Roller Coaster Sooner Than Later!

The diabetes roller coaster is the up and down (and back up) of your blood sugar. It's no fun. It's hard to stop once you're caught up in it, and it wreaks havoc on your life both mentally and physically! There's no better way to ruin a great day of plans than to find yourself caught on this roller coaster. On the flipside, though, there are things we tend to do with our insulin and food that only exacerbate the roller coaster, and there are habits we can develop to limit how often we get stuck on that ride!

Here are a few crucial tips:

1. **Whoa, take a deep breath.** If you've ever found yourself seething with frustration and anger, dealing with that up-and-down roller coaster emotionally, only to find yourself making it worse, then reminding yourself to slow down and take a deep breath *before doing anything* can save you from further anguish in the hours to come.

    Take a deep breath.

    We all feel that pressure to get our blood sugar down as quickly as possible, but it's okay if it takes an extra hour longer if that means we can prevent rebounding in the other direction, right? It's okay. And in the end, while many blood sugars seem frustratingly random, there's actually usually a very clear reason why we went low—and just because we don't have knowledge or awareness of that reason doesn't mean it doesn't exist. Human physiology is complicated! Taking more time to think clearly before acting with regard to a low or high blood sugar can save us from our impulsive behavior that may send our blood sugar raging in the opposite direction.

2. **Create a new habit around how you *think* about treating low blood sugars.** During a low, it's not that hard to let your sugar-craving brain lead you into a habit of wanting to eat everything. Everything. But that's all it is: a habit. Somewhere in your head, even though you don't *need* all the food within your reach in order to bring your low back up, you've given yourself permission to treat low blood sugars by overeating food. And that's just asking for trouble—we know that—but it's just a habit. As soon as you decide that isn't what you believe is an appropriate way to treat low blood sugars, you can start to change that habit and change the conversation in your head about what's logical and what's okay to do.

   We do have a choice. Sure, our brain is irrationally craving more, but you still have a part of your brain that's trying to remind you, "Um, logically, I do *not* actually need to eat that entire box of crackers in order to bring my blood sugar up to a safe level."

3. **Pick a few specific foods to use for treating low blood sugars.** Instead of reaching out to *any* type of food when you're low, have certain types of foods available that you chose beforehand to treat lows. For instance, I keep Gummy LifeSaver's in my car because they don't melt or freeze. I keep juice boxes in the kitchen for quick gulps. And I keep dried pineapple chunks next to my bed because *I hate having to eat in the middle of the night* and I only need one of those darn chunks of pineapple to treat a low properly. (I strive to never force feed myself a glucose tab—I just don't like 'em!) Now, I'm not saying those are the foods *you* ought to use, but the point is that you choose certain foods to be used as "medicine" and you'll therefore be less likely to overeat that food.

   We'll talk about how to enjoy treats and yummy food in the next chapter, but using a low blood sugar as an excuse to treat yourself to some ice cream rarely goes over smoothly. Personally, I'd rather enjoy some ice cream when my blood sugar is steady and I can think rationally through the accurate amount of insulin I need for the amount I ate.

Creating Goals for Diabetes Management

To give you a running start, here are a few examples of approachable goals you can create for day-to-day diabetes management:

I'm going to:

- *test my blood sugar each morning, as soon as I wake up, for 30 days.*
- *check my blood sugar six times per day on Saturdays for the next two months.*
- *pick one day each week that I will log and track my blood sugars for the next seven weeks.*
- *check off on a calendar each day that I commit to checking my blood sugar at least three times per day for the entire next month.*
- *write down one sentence each night, for a month, reflecting on what I did well in diabetes management that day.*
- *choose one meal of the day when I will carefully measure my carbohydrates for two weeks.*
- *take my vitamins and oral medications for diabetes each morning for one week while brewing my coffee.*
- *carefully calculate my insulin dose each day at lunch for two weeks and keep track of what my blood sugar was two hours after lunch to see if it was effective.*
- *choose one experiment focused on insulin doses (at meals, basal insulin, and correction insulin doses) to focus on for one entire month, then repeat for the other insulin dose options.*

With the six-step process outlined below, think about the first goal you'd like to create around your blood sugars and daily diabetes management.

1. **Understand where you're starting from.**
2. **Be super, extremely, incredibly specific.**
3. **Make sure you can measure your progress.**

4. Ask yourself *why* this matters to you.
5. Establish the tiny, supportive details.
6. Create a Pick-Up Plan.

_____

_____

_____

_____

_____

_____

_____

_____

_____

_____

_____

_____

_____

_____

_____

_____

_____

_____

What Others Have to Say

Gary Scheiner, Certified Diabetes Educator, living with type 1 diabetes
(IntegratedDiabetes.com)

It helps to work with a health care team that truly "gets it." If someone on the team has diabetes, that's a real plus. Far too often, health care providers can't relate to what it's like to live with a 24/7 condition that requires countless decisions and infinite responsibilities. It makes a big difference having someone on your health care team that you can be honest and open with about your challenges and your shortcomings.

Many patients need little more than a good cathartic venting to get themselves back on track. Health care providers need to be sympathetic and understanding, but they also need to know when to say when: a patient who is not taking their insulin, for example, is putting his life in jeopardy. There are certain "non-negotiables" when it comes to self-care.

The worst thing a health care provider can do is use "scare tactics" to try to change the behavior of someone who is burned-out. Patients know all about the ramifications of poor self-care. They don't want or need reminders, and doing so shows a complete lack of understanding of the situation.

Personally, I'm in a perpetual state of burnout! It is very difficult to spend all day helping other people with their diabetes, and then have to focus on mine as well. For a long time now, I've sort of "given up" trying to stick to a healthy meal plan. This causes blood sugar control problems for me, but I do a pretty good job in all the other areas of self-care to help make up for it.

(continued)

(continued)

What Others Have to Say

Phyllisa Deroze, living with type 2 diabetes
(DiagnosedNotDefeated.com)

I was burned-out when I was first diagnosed. In the hospital, I had to get finger pricks every two hours and receive insulin through an IV. I have experienced burnout while on insulin (it meant simply hating the finger pricks and injections, but doing it anyway); when I was on oral meds being burned-out meant skipping a dose at times. Now that I'm medicine-free, burnout looks more like not wanting to exercise because I have to. I have had more than one medical professional tell me that I don't have to check my glucose as much as I did when I was on insulin, but I can't stop. After forcing myself to go an entire week without testing, I found that I began eating horribly. Not knowing where I was before I ate caused me to eat out of proportion. So I still test daily. It's noon and I've tested my glucose three times already today. When I feel burnout, however, it means that I will test once a day.

Another challenge I find is the inability to get a handle on diabetes. While I've been a medicine-free diabetic for more than a year, I was under a lot of stress during the winter months and I could not (no matter how hard I tried) get my glucose under control. I had to take an extremely small dose of Metformin for about three months and then things were back to "my normal." I wish there was one regimen that would make managing diabetes easy. However, not only are we all different, but our diabetes is also different from day to day. One day a chocolate chip cookie fits into my carb-count perfectly, another day it causes me to spike high, and yet on another day, I could eat two without a problem.

The easiest part of diabetes management for me, usually, is counting carbs. I thrive in counting carbs. I'm a lean, mean carb-counting machine. I try my hardest to never go above 60 grams of carbs every time I eat.

(continued)

(*continued*)

What Others Have to Say

Will Dubois, diabetes educator, living with type 1 diabetes
(LifeAfterDX.blogspot.com)

I screw this up as often as I get it right. Sometimes I think my diabetes is an intelligent alien parasite. It seems like every time I do a radical therapy shake-up, I have a few really good days or weeks, but then the diabetes adapts. Blood sugar control is a real ongoing challenge for me. My averages generally work out pretty well, and I've spent my D-career mainly in the high sixes and low sevens A1C-wise, but the glycemic variation is pretty wild and that worries me. Trust me, I'm a waaaaaaay better tour guide than role model.

I don't really get burned-out, I'm not sure why. Maybe it's because I'm in the trenches helping others. I think that helps. Crazy as it sounds, it gives my diabetes, and my life, wider purpose, and that makes it easier to tolerate and accept. Ninety-eight percent of the time I really don't mind having diabetes at all, and I'm actually healthier with it than I was before I had it.

Dr. Bill Polonsky said it best: "All this hard work and your reward is that nothing bad happens." Good diabetes control has no tangible reward. That makes it hard to keep focused on good control day after day after day after day. I think people just wake up one morning and say, "F*$k this! I don't see the point."

I mean, sure, you know that keeping your blood sugar in control keeps complications at bay, but complications are monsters that live under the bed. Scary, but not quite real. The more overwhelmed you get by the effort to keep them at bay, the less real the monsters under the bed seem to be.

(*continued*)

(continued)

What Others Have to Say

What I see most commonly is people first abandoning testing of their blood sugar. I view that as the first warning sign of burnout. And then, once they aren't testing, diet awareness slips. In no time at all, people can have screaming high blood sugars and don't really realize how bad they've gotten. For the most part, patients tend to keep taking their meds. I don't too often see someone throw in the towel so much they stop their meds, but if you cut loose on your diet and don't test, your meds will be woefully inadequate.

Really, we'd be better off if high blood sugar hurt like hell. If 335 mg/dL felt like being riddled with machine gun bullets, none of us would be caught dead in a Krispy Kreme doughnut shop, right?

And one advantage of being responsible for 300 people's diabetes, not just your own, is that I'm never far from someone who's doing worse than I am. I know that sounds perverse, but if you are only aware of your own failings, that can be a lot to bear. I'm surrounded by people who fail all the time, so I know it's normal to be less than perfect, and I guess I'm not too hard on myself.

Health care workers need to understand that this is damn hard work. Most doctors have no clue what it's like to have diabetes. I often hear them complaining about "noncompliant" patients. Hey, medical school is like a walk in the park compared to diabetes. Plus, even the toughest of schools ends in graduation. Diabetes ends in death. We have no prospect of this ever being over. Of ever even getting a break from it. Sh*t, just saying this is burnin' me out!

(continued)

(continued)

What Others Have to Say

Kate Cornell, living with type 2 diabetes
(Kates-Sweet-Success.blogspot.com)

My stress level surrounding my diabetes changes constantly. In the beginning I was stressed because I had no idea what I was doing. Now, after nearly eight years, I can feel stress when my glucose levels are out of line even though I'm "doing everything right." Diabetes causes stress and frustration no matter how long you've been dealing with it.

Avoiding certain foods is definitely my biggest challenge. We've all heard that people with diabetes can eat anything, and we can to a certain extent, but those of us with T2 who don't use insulin have a tough time with high blood sugars if we don't avoid carb-heavy foods. I have identified those foods that wreak havoc with my blood sugar and I do my best to avoid them. Knowing that bread and potatoes, among other things, are bad for my glucose control doesn't make it any easier to avoid eating them.

But checking my blood sugar has never been a challenge for me. I have never complained about finger sticks, and I appreciate having this technology that helps me know how certain meals and exercise affect my glucose. There is no way I would be able to attempt to control my diabetes without it.

My burnout usually comes in the form of depression, frustration, and "woe is me" followed closely by eating all the wrong things. It's the old vicious circle: see higher numbers on the meter, try to "fix" it, fail, give up, and eat all the things in the kitchen. All that does is lead to more anxiety and higher numbers. Burnout feels like a combination of defeat and frustration with a dash of self-reproach.

(continued)

(continued)

What Others Have to Say

Sometimes I just let myself feel bad about my diabetes, but never for too long. I usually just have a talk with myself and try to remember that no one is perfect and that it's worth it to do the best I can. It's okay to visit the dark side, but it's not okay to live there.

Burnout is inevitable; how could it not be? Regardless of what your diabetes care looks like you are always reminded that not paying attention will have dire consequences down the road. Therefore, we tend to work *hard* to control diabetes without a vacation. No break = break down.

Mike Durbin, living with type 2 diabetes and congestive heart failure
(MyDiabeticHeart.com)

My life with type 2 diabetes was quite a bit different in the first several months following diagnosis than it is right now. Initially, I was put on a 1,500 calorie, low sodium diet, and the oral medication Glipizide. I was told to try to exercise as much as I could, which, given the weakened state of my heart at the time, wasn't much at all, and that I needed to lose some weight.

The combination of the dietary changes and the medications I was taking to treat the congestive heart failure led to a 30-plus pound weight loss (mostly retained fluids) in about three months and to my A1C dropping from 9.6 to 6.5 in about the same amount of time.

Frankly, though, the diet was pure hell, and often left me feeling deprived and starving most of the time. I maintained that dietary discipline for several months before reaching a point where I couldn't stand it anymore and gave up on it.

(continued)

(continued)

What Others Have to Say

Now, four and a half years later, my regimen is quite a bit different. For starters, I'm no longer following that strict 1,500-calorie diet. I didn't feel as though I was getting the nourishment I needed or felt I needed to be happy. I'm still eating a healthy diet and nutritious foods, but I'm not starving or depriving myself anymore. Moderation is the key.

And my diabetes medication regimen is quite different as well, as I made the decision to switch to injectable medications, including insulin. After struggling with medications for the last year or so, I've finally found a combination that has my A1C back at 6.5 for the first time in at least a year.

Type 2 diabetes is an incredibly challenging disease by itself, but I'm living with that, plus congestive heart failure and a few other health issues. Balancing all of them is quite difficult.

If I'm being completely honest, managing the conditions isn't the biggest challenge I face. The real challenge comes from trying to pay for everything needed to manage them. Paying for my diabetes supplies and medications, my chronic heart failure medications, hospital debts, college loans, the monthly bills, etc., is incredibly stressful and challenging. Like many, I find myself robbing Peter to pay Paul each month. I find myself having to choose between the life-sustaining medications that I need, paying the utilities, or putting food on the table. It is soul destroying to think about. Ultimately, the challenge is choosing between living life and staying alive. There is a difference.

When I'm really feeling burned-out, I tend to not pay as close attention to my daily regimen as I do when I'm on top of my game. My dietary choices aren't the best, my glucose checking becomes less frequent and, at times, I'm not as thorough with my medications as I know I need to be.

(continued)

(*continued*)

What Others Have to Say

I hate the diseases that I've been diagnosed with even more during these times. And I tend to resent the financial burdens that I face because of them, as well as resent that the life I was building for myself was stolen by them.

Allison Nimlos, living with type 1 diabetes
(TheBloodSugarWhisperer.wordpress.com)

I was diagnosed as a child, so my daily management has changed drastically overall. I would definitely say that it is much more stressful now because I'm in full control of my diabetes as compared to when I was young and relied on my parents to do most of the heavy lifting.

I have always had such a hard time remembering to test my blood sugars! It's one of the reasons I love the CGM [continuous glucose monitor] so much! I tend to zone out and lose track of time if I don't have an alarm on my phone going off to remind me to test. If it wasn't for that, I'm pretty sure I never would. I'm pretty good about testing at meals, but other tests during the day, like afternoon or even right before bed, is just something that I often forget that I need to do. I don't know if it's subconscious avoidance or what, but that's been my most consistent struggle in my management.

I've really never had an issue taking my insulin. I know how bad I feel when I forget and so I'm good about shooting up or bolusing when I eat. I'm not the greatest with carb counting, but I definitely put in the effort to bolus, and bolus the right amount. High blood sugars have such an immediate effect on how I feel, so I try to avoid high blood sugars as much as possible!

(*continued*)

(*continued*)

What Others Have to Say

When I'm burned-out then I tend to put less effort into making the necessary adjustments to my diabetes. I tend to just go on autopilot and I can have weeks of high blood sugars before I realize, "Hey! I need to change my dose!" I just avoid doing any extra thinking about my diabetes and I just do what I need to do to not die, but I don't really do anything that will actually make me healthier.

Likewise, I think it's also important to make sure your management is meeting your needs. Whether it's getting burned-out on shots, or getting tired of the pump, or needing the assistance from an app, sometimes we don't realize that the way we've been doing things just isn't working!

I think people with diabetes tend to think that we have to do everything on our own because it's our diabetes, but the truth is, our family and friends are probably more than willing to help with some of the smaller tasks in diabetes. I give my husband little things to do, like carb counting the meals he cooks, or fetching me a juice box in the middle of the night. It's not a lot, but it's a little bit, and knowing that my diabetes is shared with someone who wants me to be healthy as much as I want to be healthy really helps. You don't have to do diabetes alone.

Bethany Rose, living with type 1 diabetes
(MewithD.wordpress.com)

The most challenging aspect of diabetes management? The constant changes. I feel like I could handle diabetes a lot better if I could spend, say, a week figuring out my insulin doses and then just glide for the next year or so. Even six months. Hell, sometimes even one month would make me happy! But putting so much effort into problem solving only to have it change again from the smallest change in my life, diet, and body is the ultimate frustration for me!

(*continued*)

(*continued*)

What Others Have to Say

The easiest aspect of diabetes, for me, is testing my blood sugar. In fact, I do it way more than I need to, because I always want to know what level I am, and doing it doesn't bother me at all. (Which is funny because it's the thing nondiabetics always think they would struggle with the most.)

For me, diabetes burnout almost always involves eating things I know that I "shouldn't," or at least that aren't normally included in my diet. And almost always in larger quantities than I do include in my diet. It's like this: "Screw diabetes! Nom nom nom … ." And it usually lasts for the rest of the day, but then the next day I rein it in.

I try to catch it before it happens and put some boundaries on it. For example, if I work really hard to log my numbers prior to an endo appointment and then feel burned-out from all the thinking and tracking, I may let myself eat things I don't normally eat for the rest of the day after the appointment, but I tell myself that it's just that one day and I make myself get back on track for the next one. (And generally I do.) I also do my best not to feel guilty about it, reminding myself that I'm allowed the occasional lax day because of all the hard work I do all of the other days. Sometimes it works better than others.

Should we all anticipate some kind of burnout in life with diabetes? Oh, hell yes.

Yes, I Ate 17 Cookies, so Sue Me! 5

Becoming a Person Who Respects His or Her Body through Food

Every morsel you eat matters—especially in life with diabetes. While everyone in the world is constantly being told how important smart nutrition is, people with diabetes get an extra heap of pressure in the area of food. And by "extra heap of pressure," I really mean to say that there is a never-ending expectation that we ought to eat perfectly every day, and never, in a million years, crave anything remotely resembling a potato chip, fries, or bowl of ice cream.

And, of course, it's true, paying really close attention to how you feed your body *will* benefit your life with diabetes *tremendously*. Fact. However, the constant pressure, constant scolding from friends or family when you eat anything imperfect, and the tired phrases from your health care team, "You really need to lose weight, eat better, and exercise more," can totally and definitely backfire.

Backfire. Squash your motivation. Fill you with resentment and anger. Leave you feeling like nothing you eat is the "right thing to eat" and frustrated with your inability to avoid all the "bad foods" like a flawless diabetic machine would. Maybe you find yourself bingeing on various sugar-laden foods when no one is around, using low blood sugars as an excuse to binge on foods you usually view as forbidden, and wind up eating both thoughtlessly and purposefully in an effort to say, "%&$# you, diabetes! You cannot control me!"

This chapter is a mix of support for both the emotional challenges around food *and* some no-nonsense tips for incorporating positive changes around food into your life. I believe one of the biggest reasons we feel burnedout and frustrated around food is because we simply don't know what we are supposed to eat and what a balanced, positive life around food looks like.

I speak purely from experience when I say that aside from taking your insulin and medications, *nothing* will benefit your happiness in life with diabetes more than embracing what it means to treat your body *truly well* with food. (And exercise, of course, which we'll talk about in the next chapter!) But getting to the point where you want and know how to do that takes time, patience, and a simple desire to live a better life with diabetes.

Suddenly, All I Want Is a Chocolate Chip Cookie

I was diagnosed with celiac disease in the eighth grade about one year after my type 1 diabetes diagnosis. My very Italian family ate pasta twice a week back then, and I burst into tears in front of the doctor at the idea of no longer being able to eat spaghetti and meatballs with my brothers. (You should know, in the year 2000, the easily accessible gluten-free alternatives for things like pasta, bread, and cookies, *all* tasted like cardboard. Today's options are endless and *much* tastier.) The first thing my then-boyfriend said to me after hearing about my new diagnosis was, "*Geez*, how many diseases do you have?" (Yes, he was a real keeper!) And one of my best friends at the time immediately gasped, "Oh my gosh, I would *die* if I couldn't eat bagels!"

The thing is, for many years, I had the more "silent" kind of celiac, which simply means that even though it clearly caused harm in my body, particularly in my small intestines, I didn't have any obvious symptoms at the time of my diagnosis aside from the positive blood test and biopsy of tissue from my small intestines. This means that I could "get away with" cheating and not pay any immediate consequences. As a teenager, and on into my first three years of college, I took major advantage of this. Of course, there were months or phases during which I was more diligent about avoiding gluten, but as a whole, I cheated at least a few times a month minimum, and there were phases when I'd eat gluten almost every day in the form of bread, beer, pizza, doughnut—whatever.

And the cookies. I swear I really never cared for my mother's famously delicious chocolate chip cookies until the day a doctor told me they were suddenly off-limits. I'm just not a chocolate chip cookie kind of girl (but believe me, I love ice cream and brownies). While my brothers would all line up for the first batch of fresh cookies out of the oven, I could have cared less … until celiac came along. Then I wanted those cookies. I'd even sneak one or two from the cookie jar to avoid getting caught cheating. My parents certainly didn't come down hard on me for cheating because it was easy to say, "Well, she doesn't have any symptoms," and none of us were exceptionally educated in nutrition. But I felt guilty every time I ate gluten, and my mom worried, quietly, with an occasional raised eyebrow.

Fast-forward to the year 2007. I had spent the last three years of college eating garbage. Just garbage. A few times a week, my behavior around food could've been easily described as *bingeing*, not just eating. And while this habit didn't impact my ability to thrive in college, it was absolutely impacting my health as a young woman with two chronic illnesses through weight gain, increased insulin resistance, guilt and unhappiness, and higher blood sugars. (My A1C had been creeping up to 8.3 percent, its highest ever.)

It's really simple: I was rebelling against the rules of my celiac and my type 1 diabetes and using food as a crutch whenever I had a really stressful day. Period. Purposefully, knowingly, and consciously? Not fully, but I opened my eyes to the reality later on. I was rebelling against the restrictions, the pressure, the demands, the expectations, somewhere in the back of my head. Using food as an escape, a not-so-helpful distraction for any unhappiness or emotional situation, and abusing my body without any real benefits in return. And I felt stuck there. (Oh, don't let me forget that I had what I later realized was a symptom of celiac described as "brain fog," that left me struggling to concentrate for long periods of time!)

And then, after spending my junior year sick of feeling *so sick*, I started going to the gym and teaching myself the basics of weightlifting through books. I went to Ashtanga yoga classes on the days between weightlifting, and by the end of that summer, I'd lost 15 pounds, gained noticeable muscle definition in my arms and legs, and reduced my background insulin dose about 10 units due to the increase in insulin sensitivity. Oh, and I stopped eating gluten—I just stopped. Most importantly, my head felt clear—goodbye brain fog. Food was no longer a weapon or a temporary distraction. It was something I used to genuinely respect and fuel my body. And that was an incredible new feeling.

But it wasn't until I hired a personal trainer, Andrew, at the gym where I later became a personal trainer and yoga instructor myself, that I truly began to learn about how much was possible through smart nutrition and exercise. You see, Andrew and two of the other trainers at the gym, Norm and Beth, were bodybuilders. Now, bodybuilding really *never* intrigued me; I was far more fascinated by the strength gained from lifting rather than the appearance gained by lifting. But I was in awe as I learned that these bodybuilders put more energy into counting their carbohydrates than I certainly ever had in the past several years for the sake of my diabetes.

They didn't *have* to watch what they ate because of some disease. They just did it for the sake of their sport, and their health. They actually *chose* to count carbs. This was a perspective on food I had forgotten was even an option after spending so many years wrapped up in eating things simply because someone told me I shouldn't. And *this* perspective on food was totally liberating, because it was a choice, *My choice.*

You see, I believe one of the most detrimental and most common beliefs we form about food and life with diabetes, is that "other people don't have to watch what they eat because they don't have diabetes." This belief fuels our resentment for food, and fuels our justification in ignoring how important it is that we feed our bodies well. But most importantly, the belief that other people don't have to pay attention to how they eat is simply not true. Sure, the impact of our choices about food tend to be immediately obvious through our blood sugar levels—which is the primary source of the pressure we feel to be perfect—but *everyone* would benefit from eating more healthy foods and less sugar. Everyone would benefit from being aware of how many carbohydrates they're consuming each day. Everyone would benefit from exercising more often. Everyone.

Embracing that fact, and letting go of the resentment many of us have felt toward people who don't have diabetes is one of the most freeing and positive things we can do for ourselves. Embracing this in my own life has changed *everything* about food and exercise, and everything about my attitude toward managing my diabetes. Everything. It has led me to feeling confident, proud, and passionate about the way I take care of my health.

And better yet, through taking better care of myself I have surrounded myself with friends who care about their own health just as much. Have you ever tried making positive changes in how you eat only to find your friends trying to sabotage your efforts because they're simply jealous they aren't making those same changes in their own lives? When you surround yourself with people who live healthy lives, you don't feel like the oddball skipping the side of fries and ordering a side of broccoli instead, or trading a late cocktail at your favorite bar for getting to bed so you can wake up early for your morning cardio session—because all of your friends are doing the same thing.

Working my way from someone who used food as a weapon for self-sabotage to someone who *loves* making positive choices about food and craves real exercise was a natural and gradual process that has completely eliminated any stress or woe about food and exercise.

And I want to share that process with you.

Your Diabetes Relationship with Food

Thinking back as far as you can, maybe even to *before* your diabetes diagnosis, can you recall who and what has shaped the way you behave around food? We learn about food through our parents, our siblings, our friends, the television, magazines, and, of course, the Internet. And we don't just learn the good stuff. From all of those sources, we can learn how to overeat food, obsess about food, feel guilty about food, hide food, and use food as a reward or a temporary escape from our emotions. If you're struggling with food in your life today, it's possible that some of the habits or beliefs you have about food stemmed from something you learned from someone or somewhere else. Sometimes, the very simple act of realizing and acknowledging why and what you're doing around food is enough to trigger a major change, but it takes a level of honesty with yourself in order to see the truth. Other times, realizing what's causing your behavior around food is just one step of the process.

Here are a few of the common signs of a self-destructive relationship with food:
- You try to eat as little as possible during the day and find yourself overeating at night to compensate for how hungry you are
- You use food regularly to comfort an emotion or avoid certain feelings such as fear, stress, anger, sadness, loneliness, guilt, and pain
- You feel ashamed or embarrassed by your secret behavior around food

- You sabotage your own health purposefully to punish yourself
- You eat very carefully in public, but feel out of control when you're eating in private
- You're convinced you have no willpower or self-control
- You use food constantly to reward yourself for just about anything
- You try to avoid certain types of foods, and binge on them uncontrollably when they are around
- You are constantly thinking about, stressed about, and worrying about food
- You regularly engage in strict fad dieting, always trying to completely eliminate entire food groups only to find yourself bingeing on those foods after a short period of time

Maybe you've become so used to some or all of these behaviors that you've convinced yourself they're sort of normal, and everyone else exhibits these behaviors, too. Maybe you're convinced that you'll never be able to change these behaviors, or can't imagine any other way of handling your emotions or your stress other than abusing your body with food simply because you've been doing this for so long.

The term "crash-dieting" certainly doesn't apply only to people with diabetes, but because of the endless pressure we are always under to lose weight and eat perfectly, it's easy to hope that the next fad-diet is the answer to all your troubles around food. The problem with most fad-diets is that they aren't structured in a way that you can actually follow in the long-term. You're bound to feel like you've failed on a strict, fad-diet. And the endless cycle of signing up for crash-diet after crash-diet absolutely leads to tremendous burnout about food and diabetes as a whole.

Here are a few things to know about conventional "dieting:"

- Losing weight extremely quickly is *not* an effective, long-term solution to lifelong maintenance of your weight. You probably already know this! Instead, put your head in the right frame of mind to embrace a 1- to 2-pound weight-loss per week as true success.
- Crash-dieting becomes a self-destructive cycle because you're bound to fail if it's too strict to maintain for long. If you're on a diet plan that leaves you feeling really, really hungry, then you are *not* on a long-term,

sustainable nutrition plan! Instead, focus on choosing a *lifestyle* approach toward nutrition that promotes good choices rather than promoting extremely fast weight-loss, strict rules, or extreme calorie reductions. A *lifestyle* approach toward eating is about eating higher-quality foods, and replacing highly processed foods with more *real* foods.

- Starving your metabolism with a low-calorie, super-strict diet will not help you lose weight and it *will* stunt your metabolism! One of the simplest ways to prevent binge-eating late at night is to *eat* more satiating food during the day—literally, eat *more* good food, and less diet food.
- Diets often expect 100 percent perfection even though we know the human brain can only sustain a certain amount of willpower for so long. Whatever *lifestyle* of eating you choose, make sure it includes treats (really high-quality treats) and doesn't demand 100 percent perfection.

In reality, you are the only one who can decide when enough is enough, but we have to start by acknowledging what's really going on in your head that is driving any particular behavior. On our own, we tend to skip over this part and just commit ourselves to a crazy diet program, like using duct-tape to fix the broken handle on your refrigerator door: that's only going to last for so long before the handle falls off again!

Now, it's your turn.

What self-destructive habits or beliefs about food and nutrition have you possibly learned from a family member, friend, or magazine?

Example: Eat as few calories as possible until you are so hungry you wind up binge-eating for days.

_____

_____

_____

_____

_____

_____

_____

_____

_____

_____

And then of course, we need to add diabetes to that mix—a disease that is obsessive about food. *Obsessive.* You can't talk about any type of diabetes without talking about food and weight and exercise. Unfortunately, those conversations about food often revolve around what you *shouldn't* or *can't* eat, rather than focusing on the many, many other things there are to eat. (Of course, there's also the problem of getting inaccurate or outdated information on nutrition that leaves you feeling even more constricted, like old-fashioned theories that eating fat makes you fat). All of the above can lead to major resentment and self-destructive behavior.

The major bummer is that the more we pretend the way we feed and exercise our body doesn't matter, and the more we pretend that our diabetes doesn't matter, the more obtrusive diabetes becomes in our life. The more we feel lethargic and depressed with high blood sugars. The more we gain weight that leads to insulin resistance, higher blood sugars, and even more weight gain. The more we pretend that our actions don't matter, the more this disease interrupts every other part of life: work, friends, relationships, family—you name it.

Describe what your current behavior and relationship with food looks like today:

_____

_____

_____

_____

_____

Is your behavior around food driven by resentment or an effort to rebel against your diabetes? If not, then what drives your decisions and behavior around food?

_____

_____

_____

_____

_____

Chances are, you've gone down the route of trying to improve your habits around food before. And chances are, there are a few things you've done that really weren't effective, and a few things you *keep* doing even though they weren't effective the first time.

Make a list of the things you've already tried to improve your behavior and choices around food that *have not* worked for you:

Example: Trying to go six months without eating any sugar … which made me feel obsessed with sugar within two weeks!

_____

_____

_____

_____

_____

_____

_____

_____

Now take a really good moment to stare at this list, and promise yourself that you won't waste another moment trying to use any of these approaches, fast-fixes, crash-dieting tactics, or denial strategies to improve your relationship with food. You already know they don't work well for you. And that brings you one step closer to ending the cycle of feeling totally frustrated and burned-out around food.

There's Definitely a Time and Place for Ice Cream … but This Isn't It

Okay, so tell me, does it *lessen or intensify* the emotion when you abuse an entire bag of chips and half a pint of ice cream? Do you feel better … or worse? Do you feel less stressed out or less upset or less angry at your diabetes? Do you feel like diabetes isn't controlling you anymore when you're full of Chinese food and three doughnuts and a bottle of soda?

Probably not. Right? But I totally, completely understand how you got there, because the pressure to do it all perfectly is so freaking annoying and it never goes away. And that's a fact. Now *because* that's a fact, what if you decided to ignore that pressure? I don't mean ignore it and eat garbage quality food mindlessly, but actually take several steps back—*way back*—and look at what life would be like *without* diabetes. If you *didn't* have diabetes, wouldn't it still be just as important that you treated your body respectfully with food? If you *didn't* have diabetes, wouldn't it still be logical and reasonable to view things like cupcakes or ice cream or pizza as an occasional treat rather than something you'd eat every day? And if you *didn't* have diabetes, would overeating food in an effort to comfort your emotions be just as ineffective and self-destructive?

Take a step way back and look at what's possible through making choices about food. Period. Diabetes doesn't even have to be a part of it. If you spend two minutes at lunch with my best friend, Tara—who has no existing health issues—you'll see someone who is incredibly meticulous about how she feeds her body. *And* she loves the food she eats! Her focus on the food she eats doesn't come from pressure from doctors or family members because of a disease (and actually, she has family and friends who try to sabotage her healthy habits all the time merely out of jealousy). Instead, the energy she puts into her nutrition each day comes purely out of her desire to live a long, healthy life.

Imagine, if you made choices about food regardless of your diabetes but simply because you wanted to take good care of your body? Because you respect your body? Because you appreciate your body?

Literally, close your eyes and envision the difference.

Willpower vs. Becoming a Person Who Respects His or Her Body through Food

Traditional dieting usually goes hand-in-hand with words like "willpower" and "discipline" and unspoken words like "deprivation." But willpower on its own has never been the successful answer for those who find lifelong changes in how they behave around food, because research has shown us clearly that willpower *does* run out! Our brains can literally only handle so much self-restraint for so long.

What if, instead, the changes in your relationship with food were motivated and fueled by a personal evolution? Something much deeper than just wanting to lose weight and trying to avoid dessert. That evolution may be gradual—it certainly doesn't have to happen overnight—but it implies that you have literally become someone who no longer engages in certain types of self-destructive behavior around food simply because you now have different beliefs around food.

Think of those persons in your life who have tremendous "discipline" about what they eat, and ask yourself, "Are they constantly trying to restrain themselves from food or are they simply following a set of beliefs they've created in their life that help guide them to make better decisions about food?"

There's a big difference.

One approach involves constantly fighting with yourself. The other involves developing knowledge and awareness about your own perspective on food.

For example, in my own life, you could sit me down in front of a fast food chain's double cheeseburger, a big strawberry shake, and some fries,

I would very easily be able to say, "No, thanks," even though I love strawberry ice cream and cheeseburgers. Why? Because I have a very strong personal belief that fast food isn't something I want in my body. Now, I would gladly make room in my week for a grass-fed organic cheeseburger and some very high-quality strawberry ice cream, but I'm also someone who believes those kinds of foods are meant to be treats, and therefore only occur on special occasions, rather than viewing them as just another meal of the day.

Developing these types of beliefs in your own life takes time, learning, and practice, but most of all, you'll want to take a step back and ask yourself, "What kinds of beliefs do I want in my life concerning food and how I feed my body?"

What would a positive relationship with food in life with diabetes look and feel like to you?

What kinds of beliefs would you like to develop about food? Be as specific as you can!

Example: A positive relationship, in my opinion, would include both discipline and flexibility. I wouldn't expect myself to be so rigid or strict that I felt deprived, but I would make a conscious and continuous effort to make decisions about food based on what I know is good for my body throughout 80 percent of the day. I would make choices based on self-respect and knowledge, rather than on impulse or emotion.

_____

_____

Now ask yourself, what's stopping you from making the above statement your reality?

_____

_____

_____

_____

_____

_____

_____

Now take a look at your answer. Is the obstacle keeping you from achieving your ideal relationship with food something that's in your power to change? If the answer is "Yes," then the next question to ask is *why*. Why are you allowing that obstacle to keep you from achieving your goals related to food? Most likely, it circles back to the not-so-helpful coping habits we discussed in Chapter 2. Somehow, your current habits around food are serving a purpose in your life that you may be afraid to let go of.

And lastly, just how tired and sick are you of letting this obstacle stand in your way?

_____

_____

_____

_____

_____

_____

_____

_____

_____

When you make a choice, when you decide you've had enough and you're tired of letting that obstacle get in the way, you are the one who makes the change. Simple, yes? Yup. One of the most empowering and yet overwhelming realities we face in life with diabetes is that we get to make the decisions. Learning *how* to make those decisions, though, can be the hardest part! For instance, can a person with diabetes ever *decide* to enjoy dessert and not feel guilty about it afterwards? You bet. In fact, let's start there…

Something Sweet or Something Salty! Yum

Let's take all the crazy drama and guilt out of sweet or greasy treats by talking about how to include them in your life. Usually, in diabetes or nutrition books, the part about dessert or junk food treats comes at the end, but I'm gonna cut right to the chase and talk about when and where the not-so-healthy food fits in. (Don't worry, we'll talk about the *healthy* foods in the next section, but this is important!) You see, a positive relationship with food does not mean you must be *perfect* and avoid all things containing sugar, grease, or salt.

Wait, I just want to make sure you really read that clearly. Allow me to repeat: a positive relationship with food *does not mean you must be perfect.*

Striving for perfection around food is bound to make anyone crazy, whether their natural cravings steer them toward Al's French Fry Stand or Wanda's Double-Dipped Chocolate Fudge Cake. Ask any competitive bodybuilder or super-fit actress or Sylvester Stallone, and they'll tell you: they always make room for treats. They *plan* to eat treats. And it actually supports their goals in health and weight-loss. Learning how to indulge, how to enjoy a "treat" food now and then is a crucial part of learning how to live well with diabetes around food.

I'm telling you, there's gotta be room in your life for an occasional treat. That treat may be every other day or once a week or just on the weekends, but it's gotta be there—even if, in your opinion, a treat is a really expensive French cheese with the world's best prosciutto, you are treating yourself to something you wouldn't normally buy or eat. And most importantly, you need to remind yourself that it's okay! It's okay to enjoy a few cookies or a really delicious snack of greasy pepperoni. It's okay to go out with your girl-friend for ice cream. *It's okay.*

There is a *big* difference between overeating a dessert or a treat during an impulsive, emotional, and out-of-control moment versus making the thoughtful decision that "I'm going to enjoy a treat today," and enjoying that treat while keeping a close eye on your blood sugar, rather than trying to ignore it.

Think of it this way: if you expect yourself to *never* eat a treat ever again, you'll inevitably find yourself bingeing on that treat, continuing that emotional cycle and negative relationship with food. However, if you make room in your life for those treats in a balanced and reasonable way, you can remove the guilt and emotion and simply enjoy every bite.

Should Your House Contain Zero Treats or Lots of Treats?

There are definitely two ways to approach how you decide to include treats in your life. The first approach is to clear them out of your house entirely, and therefore the only time you enjoy a treat is when you actually get up and leave your house to go find that treat. The theory here is that the getting up and going out part will sway you from actually getting a treat. My personal feeling on this approach is that it only instills the obsession for whatever that food is. And by the time you do get it in your hands, you're much more likely to binge on it because it's been kept from you for whatever length of time.

This approach, I feel, actually magnifies and encourages binge eating and negative relationships with treat foods.

The second approach, and the one I use with my coaching clients, is to actually stock up on whatever treat item you love the most. Using ice cream as an example, I would actually recommend that you buy so many pints of Ben & Jerry's ice cream that there's no way you could possibly eat it all in one sitting. (And yes, you'll notice I did *not* suggest you buy some unsatisfying, yucky, low-calorie, low-fat ice cream that simply leaves you craving *real* ice cream later on. If you're gonna have a treat, have a *real* treat that actually tastes great and is worth the calories!)

Many people fear having a pint of really good ice cream in their freezer because they're convinced they can't possibly restrain themselves from eating the whole darn thing, but that is just a mindset, just something you've been telling yourself, and something you're encouraging by avoiding the ice cream and then buying it on an impulse. Instead, pick one treat food and buy a bunch of it. Maybe you over-do it the first couple nights and eat too much, but I guarantee, at a certain point, that food item isn't going to be so darn powerful and have so much control over you after a week or two.

If you're nervous about the second approach, then try both for a couple of weeks, and see what happens. Most people have already tried the first approach many times in their life with little to no avail, and wind up telling me things like, "Oh, I can't have that in my house! I go crazy for it!" My response to that is, "Actually, if that food really has *that* much control over your behavior that implies to me that you should definitely put a lot of it in your house so you can truly get over that behavior!"

Suddenly, you just might find that food you've felt helpless around for your whole life is not such a big deal, because it's *always* there. And you won't be telling anymore horror stories about how such-and-such food ruined your weekend and made you sick after you ate 14 servings.

Structuring Your Treats to Suit Your Current Life

Everyone is different—especially when it comes to how many treats each week is appropriate for them or how those treats ought to be structured throughout the week. In my own life, for example, I've gone through phases where it felt best to keep my treats structured more carefully to happen just on the weekends, or even *just* on Sundays. I found the structure to be helpful and supportive in keeping me focused on my other nutritional goals during the rest of the week.

There have been other phases in the past several years, when I genuinely felt most balanced when I treated myself every single day, but I compensated for that daily treat by cutting back my carbohydrate intake elsewhere in the day. Literally, this means I made room for Ben & Jerry's ice cream by not eating any carbohydrates at breakfast or dinner because I knew I felt best when I consumed between 50 and 75 grams of carbohydrates per day and I wanted to keep myself in that range while still enjoying some ice cream.

Lately, my desire for sweet things has been truly minimal. So I don't plan my treat meals at all, because when I do start craving something a little sweet, it's once or twice a week and I don't need much of it to feel satisfied.

And that brings me to the difference between your past life of using food as a self-destructive tool and the treat meals of your future: treat meals do not blatantly sabotage your health or leave you feeling guilty and ashamed. Instead, treat meals are sized appropriately. Treat meals include carb-counting and careful doses of insulin. And treat meals come with balance. If you know you're going to indulge in the carbohydrates from fries at your best friend's bachelor party this weekend, then balance your day by reducing the carbohydrates you eat earlier in the day. When you take the emotion out of it, and just approach the treat logically, it can be simple *and* much more enjoyable!

Tips for structuring your treats:

- If you are currently struggling with bingeing on sweets or salty things when you're restricted from them, then I would recommend you start by planning a treat once a day or once every other day at the least. Over the course of a few weeks, you can start to gradually cut back after the newness of having the freedom to enjoy a treat has worn off, especially if weight-loss is one of your primary goals.
- If you are someone who is already on the path to more mindful eating habits and finding success in filling your body with more real and whole

foods, think about how often you genuinely crave something sweet, and just aim to satiate that craving in a moderate, thoughtful way a few times a week.

- If you are someone who genuinely loves structure, has a very busy week but a not so busy weekend, then giving yourself the freedom to eat what you want on Saturday and/or Sunday, within appropriate amounts, might be a great fit for you.

The key is: put some careful thought into what *really* makes sense for your life right now. If you have never tried to change your eating habits and food choices, then trying to be perfect *all* week long is probably not a very smart idea. But if you feel as if you've already done a lot of the groundwork around your eating habits, then spreading your treats out accordingly can work well.

Remember, the treat is *not* a reward for eating perfectly during the week or for getting promoted at work or winning a free vacation to the Bahamas. Puppies get rewards for learning how to sit and be cute. You are not a puppy. You are a human who is learning how to respect your body with a balanced lifestyle around food, and that balanced lifestyle simply includes some treats.

Random Foods That Make My Blood Sugar Act a Fool!

One of the very best things we can each do is identify which types of carbohydrates throw our blood sugars out of control more than others—and weirdly enough, this has little to do with how "healthy" the food is, and more to do with simply our own individual bodies.

For instance, not only does oat*meal* make me just feel like total "bleh" in the morning, but it also seems to never accept my usual insulin-to-carbohydrate ratio that works very well for oat*bran*—which makes me feel ready to rock 'n' roll in the morning. And yet, balancing my blood sugar around a bowl of full-fat Ben & Jerry's ice cream is like child's play for me. I am the master of my domain with a bowl of ice cream, always finding myself at 135 mg/dL after a mere three-unit dose.

The five most common foods I hear folks struggling with are high-fat/high-carb combos:

1. pizza
2. Chinese food
3. sushi
4. cereal
5. ice cream

Oh, grapes. Grapes are so good. So tasty. But man alive, I can never get the carb-count right with those damn juicy treats! No matter how closely I try to measure and count and dose along with the weirdly large amount of insulin I take for a mere bowl of grapes, I always wind up with a blood sugar between 200 and 300 mg/dL an hour later.

Sushi? I know I'm not alone when it comes to sushi. I've read in places (that I cannot find for you today) that the process of cooking sushi rice increases the amount of glucose/starch on each grain of rice. I can't prove this, I just know I've read it somewhere, and it helps me feel better about the impossible high blood sugars I always seem to have after eating sushi.

While I only find myself at a sushi restaurant maybe twice per year, I've decided personally that it just isn't worth the high blood sugars anymore and I aim to stick to sashimi and seaweed salads at any future Japanese dining events. I don't, however, plan to stop eating grapes; instead, I just know I need to check my blood sugar a lot shortly after eating them and thus take more insulin. They're too yummy to quit.

And cereal, honestly, I keep a box of gluten-free Chex stuffed way back in my pantry *purely* for moments when I know my blood sugar is bottoming out in a severe kind of way—one of those lows where you know you have way too much insulin on board and the idea of chugging a whole jug of juice feels nauseating—that's when I eat cereal.

Chinese food makes its way to my belly about one to two times per year, and I simply aim to avoid the rice, take a good amount of insulin for the sugar in all of the sauces that I can't possibly measure, and check my blood sugar often after the meal to stay on top of any creeping highs.

My point is simply that some foods, for you or for me, can make our blood sugars act *extra* crazy. Sure, *any* food containing carbohydrates or large amounts of protein will raise our blood sugar without fine-tuned insulin doses, but some foods seem to have an extra BOOM impact. Maybe you're master of your domain when it comes to grapes—that's cool—'cause everybody's different.

If you're striving for better blood sugars, then pinpointing exactly which foods are extra troublesome for you—and then limiting those foods in your life—can be tremendously helpful. Like I said, I love cereal, but I choose *never* to eat it unless it's low blood sugar *emergency*. Otherwise, the blood sugar roller coaster headache that follows a bowl of cereal (or a plate of sushi) just isn't worth it.

That's all.

Not So Sugar-Coated: Then What the Heck Should I Eat?

I want to start this off by pointing out that you *CAN* actually eat whatever you want. *No one* is forcing food down your throat and no one is going to send you to jail for eating a doughnut or fast food or a huge bowl of the most sugary cereal in the grocery store. You are the only one who is truly in charge of how you feed your body, which means you *choose* how you feed your body. In the end, my simple hope for you is that you won't let the emotions and pressures around life with diabetes choose for you. Instead, coming to a place in your life where you make thoughtful decisions about food, whether it's a treat or a bowl full of steamed vegetables, will give you freedom, peace of mind, and empowerment in your life with diabetes around food.

Okay, now onto the food:

I'm going to bring this up again, and again because it's *that* important: forget about diet programs and forget the number on the scale—especially for the first three to six months that you start working on your nutrition. Forget about calorie counting or low-fat, low-calorie diet foods. Instead, focus on filling your plate with *more* REAL food rather than the stuff that comes in a box or a package or a wrapper. (This means most of your grocery store items will come from the outside aisles in the store, rather than inside on the shelves.) What should you eat? Real food! Start eating more real food. Period. This is the number one most simple thing you could ever do for your life in relation to food and your life with diabetes.

Now, you're probably thinking, "Well, what about bread? Isn't bread a real food?" Well, not really. Bread is a really *common* food, but if you read the list of ingredients in your bread, are there any ingredients in there that you can't pronounce because they're a chemical, rather than a food item? If you're gonna get your carb-intake from bread, make sure it's *real* bread. Great quality bread. Or, better yet, get your carbohydrates from things like quinoa, whole oats and oat bran, sweet potatoes, and brown rice. Real, whole foods that haven't been mixed together with a variety of preservatives and chemicals.

What about something like almond milk? Well, sure, almond milk was processed because someone had to soak the almonds to create the milk, but as far as "milk" products go, you can't go wrong with a glass of unsweetened almond milk.

So clearly there's some flexibility in what is considered "processed" versus "real" food. And nobody said you had to avoid *all processed foods*. I'm talking about simply increasing your consumption of real food. Increasing your interest in preparing and cooking real food for meals instead of eating fast food or prepackaged microwave dinners. I'm talking about filling your body with more of the real stuff, so you have less room in your belly for the overly processed stuff.

It's that simple, for the basics. Seriously. Real food. Are you sick of hearing that yet? Now, let's get down to business and talk about how you can take your ambitious efforts to improve your nutrition to the next level— when you're ready!

Top 10 *Effective* Tips for Improving Your Eating Habits

The following tips are *not* sugar-coated. While we've talked a lot in this chapter about the emotional challenges around nutrition, there's another side to that story: the way we feed our bodies absolutely impacts how well we thrive in life with diabetes. If we continue to eat crumby, junky food, we will continue to struggle even more with our health and our blood sugars. If we choose to make improvements, bit-by-bit, in the choices we make about food, we will reap the benefits. But that "making improvements" is a process, and it doesn't necessarily happen in a few months or even a few years. For many, it's an ongoing evolution! But the fact is that food does matter, and caring about what you eat *does not* have to mean you're deprived or stressed by every decision.

In my own life, as I've mentioned, I take my own nutrition very seriously, but I wasn't always that way about food. Actually, looking back, I ate pretty horribly up until my third year of college. And then, looking back just on the few years after that where I *was* trying very hard to improve how I was eating, I know today that much of what I thought was a "healthy diet" was still really lacking. There are *many* ways to eat healthfully and feed your body well. Whether you're vegan, low-carbing, high-carbing—whatever—there is still a basis of quality and care that goes into your choices about food. And that starts with knowledge, experimenting, and practice!

Today, I know that my body, my energy, my blood sugars, and my weight feel *optimum* and *awesome* when I eat a gluten-free and low-to-moderate carbohydrate diet of less than 100 grams of carbohydrates per day that consists mostly of: organic veggies, beans, and fruits; grass-fed and organic meats such as steak, pork, chicken, fish, and nitrate-free bacon; minimal dairy (i.e., the occasional slice of cheese or brie on rice crackers); healthy fats from nut butters, coconut oil and olive oil, almond milk, and organic eggs; grains like oat bran, quinoa, and brown rice; egg-white protein powder; minimal artificial sweeteners coming only from plant-based sources like xylitol and stevia; and last but not least, occasional treats that are made with care and quality, like *really* great ice cream or maple fudge or a gluten-free brownie I made at home.

I love food. I don't feel stressed out by food *ever* anymore. And I feel empowered on a daily basis through the way I feed my body. But like I said, that process came with a lot of practice, learning, experimenting, and more learning! Over the course of at least *four years*.

To add another perspective on the same note, my good friend Riva Greenberg, who has lived with type 1 diabetes for over 40 years (and authored many books about living well with this ol' disease), describes her own evolution with food: "I've grown to love healthy foods over the years and I eat exactly what I like: oatmeal for breakfast with seeds and nuts and Greek yogurt. Grilled chicken over salad for lunch. Usually fish or chicken for dinner with low starch vegetables and maybe beans. I snack on nuts, eat dark chocolate at night for my sweet tooth. I don't crave sweets or scones or bagels anymore. And when I want a few bites of my husband's tiramisu or I want fried calamari or whatever, I have it. For me, nothing's off limits, but 85 percent of the time I eat healthy because I like it, and I like knowing it's keeping me healthy. And, let me tell you, I was a teenager who squashed lots of lonely feelings with Ring Dings and Drake's coffee cakes."

It's a gradual evolution of wanting mostly great things for your body and feeling good about the small percentage of treats you enjoy.

The following tips are straightforward suggestions about nutrition *if* you are someone who *wants* to learn and improve the way you eat. If you aren't ready for that step, and still working on the emotional aspects of your relationship with food, then these tips might be helpful later on down the road.

1. Pick One Part of the Day to Focus on First

For some people, changing their entire nutritional life all at once can work very well, but for many, it's really overwhelming and ineffective. Instead of trying to change everything you're eating, spend a few weeks just trying to make better choices at breakfast, or in the evening. After you've tackled that part of the day and maintained some consistency, you can start to focus on another part of the day's nutrition. For example, if you've been eating a standard commercialized cereal for breakfast (which tend to be packed with added sugars, artificial flavors, and a variety of ingredients that don't look like food), focus on transitioning to taking the time to make yourself a few eggs with a bowl of oat bran instead. Nutritional changes don't have to happen all at once in order to qualify as progress!

Another very important thing to remember is that if you suddenly decide to reduce the carbohydrates in your diet, that means you need to *increase* your intake from other sources, specifically fat and protein. If you don't, you'll find yourself stuck with egg whites and spinach at breakfast, and starving barely an hour later. This is the number one most common struggle I see in those who try to reduce their carbs—they forget to increase their fat intake! Don't be afraid of eating more fat if you're working hard to reduce the processed carbohydrates in your diet.

2. Lose That Fear of the Kitchen and Cooking!

Improving how you eat will never happen if you don't get over your fear of cooking. It can be *so* easy without requiring hours in the kitchen and bizarre ingredients you've never heard of. (Trust me, I do not cook fancy recipes, but I prepare fresh veggies and fresh protein each night for dinner without much effort.) Find a basic cooking class in your area so you can discover how simple it is to simply sauté, roast, bake, grill, steam, or boil fresh ingredients such as veggies and lean protein. You don't need a lot of ingredients, just a good olive or coconut oil for cooking, a variety of simple herbs or spices, and your options are endless.

In my own life, I consider myself to be a pretty lazy cook, but I eat fresh, whole foods every single night. For example, I choose a raw vegetable (my faves are fresh broccoli, bell peppers, asparagus, onions, and frozen peas or corn), and a source of great quality protein, like grass-fed meat or organic chicken or fish. I brush a light layer of coconut oil on the meat or veggies, sprinkle a variety of herbs or spices on top and grill, or sauté for up to 15 minutes. (Baking and broiling takes a bit longer, and I don't have that much patience). Some days of the week, I might also make quinoa, cooked in vegetable bouillon, mixed with frozen peas and corn. Delicious and so simple. Now, that might not fit into your dietary likings, but over the years I've experimented with a variety of strategies about food and discovered what supports my energy and my diabetes best.

The point is, though, that cooking does *not* have to be a big fancy thing in order to be healthy. Get over your fear of learning how to cook, ask a skillful friend or relative to help, watch countless hours of Ellie Krieger or Martha Stewart (or whatever!) and *build your skills in the kitchen!*

3. Never Stop Educating Yourself about Nutrition

The more you learn about what you're putting into your body and how it impacts every part of your health, the more easily you will be convinced to avoid the processed junk and choose the right stuff. But beware, there are a lot of outdated nutritional guidelines out there (like eggs, for example, which were falsely given a bad reputation a long time ago), so it's time to start learning. When your decisions about food come from your own education, rather than someone *telling* you what you should or shouldn't eat, the way you behave around food becomes empowering, instead of stressful or ridden with guilt.

Right now, I want you to download two podcasts on your phone or your computer so you can start learning about the real sciences of nutritional research. Easy to understand and convincingly straightforward, check out Abel James's "The Fat-Burning Man," and Jimmy Moore's "Livin' La Vida Low Carb." I also highly recommend anything from Dr. Mark Hyman about nutrition through his books or articles on the Internet.

After enough learning on the topic, I chose to stop consuming artificial sweeteners except for the plant-based natural sweeteners (stevia and xylitol), which I only consume in my protein powder after strength-training workouts. A year before that, though, I was consuming artificial sweeteners like sucralose and aspartame *all the time* and I didn't care. Removing those sweeteners from my diet was a choice I made on my own.

4. Make the Choice to Want Good Things for Your Body

Instead of feeling that you need to care about what you eat while "other people can eat whatever they want," realize that you are *choosing* to make decisions about nutrition for your own benefit. No one is forcing this upon you—literally, you're the one who puts the food in your mouth! And whether or not someone else has diabetes doesn't mean that what they eat won't impact their own health, too. I *don't* eat healthfully because someone told me I have to; I eat healthfully because I *want* and *choose* to eat those foods. I love the way I feel when I treat my body a certain way. I love the energy

I have when my food choices help my blood sugar goals, and my choices about food came from my own beliefs about what I want to feed my body.

Of course, when I was younger, this definitely wasn't the case. I worked to get to that point in my relationship with food. During my first two years of college, I ate whatever I felt like eating (especially gluten and plenty of desserts), and as a result my A1C was higher, I gained weight, and my energy and self-esteem were definitely lacking. When I finally let go of the resentment for being told I couldn't eat gluten and shouldn't eat candy, I was able to make choices based entirely on my desire to be healthier and happier.

5. Read the Ingredients

Sure, diabetics are told to count carbohydrates and calories, but if you haven't taken a look at the list of ingredients in everything you eat, you're in for a big surprise. How many of those words actually look like *food*? If you can't pronounce it and have no idea what it is, why would you want it in your body? Aiming to consume more *real foods* and less of the processed stuff the food industry has created to make food cheaper to produce will inevitably improve your overall nutritional lifestyle. Have you ever read the ingredients on the back of *everything* you ate? Give it a try.

Remember, just because something says it "only contains 100 calories" doesn't mean it's actually a *healthy* food. Instead, it just means it's 100 calories, but what kinds of ingredients make up those 100 calories? Real food, or a variety of chemicals and preservatives? Personally, I'd rather treat myself to a really delicious homemade, gluten-free, no-bake chocolate cookie than some store-bought, low-fat, low-calorie, yucky diet dessert that only has 100 calories because there isn't any *real* food in it! And the yummy homemade treat will be much more satisfying!

6. Fewer Excuses, More Thoughtful Choices

I've heard a million and more excuses about not being able to eat healthier foods. "If I actually cook things myself, then I'll have to wash the dirty dishes." Yes, welcome to the world where we all have to clean our own dishes. "It's hard to keep vegetables fresh in the fridge." Except, if you eat them every night, they shouldn't be sitting in the fridge all week, right? "It takes so much time to cook eggs in the morning." Cracking and cooking two eggs into a hot pan takes less than five minutes—I do it almost every morning.

I'm gonna put this bluntly: if you care about your health and are trying to be healthier, then you'll never step into a fast food joint ever again except to use the bathroom during a long drive! There's no *real* food in there, and there are *always* other choices. During a road-trip, you can just as easily go to a grocery store as you can to a fast food restaurant. Buy a combination of fresh fruit, mixed nuts, veggies and hummus, or even a freshly made sandwich with lean deli-meats. Sure, the grocery store meal will cost more than a 99-cent burger, but why do we spend more money on our smartphones and clothing than we're willing to spend on the food we put in our bodies?

And yes, if you *want* to eat fast food regularly, then no one can stop you—it's your choice—but there certainly is no shortage of books and documentaries exposing the reality of how detrimental it is to your life.

If you're struggling to find healthy choices at lunch during your workday, consider making extra food at dinner the night before to bring with you. Put that extra quantity of food immediately into a lunch-sized container and it'll be waiting for you the next morning. Yes, this requires a little bit of planning, but your health is *worth it*.

There are a million excuses, but as soon as you make your health an actual priority, those excuses are meaningless.

7. Learn How to Count Carbohydrates

As obnoxious as this is, it's a major reality for anyone living with diabetes (and is just as helpful for people who *don't* live with diabetes, actually). When you're ready and feeling motivated to focus on nutrition, grab a little notebook or a fancy app on your smartphone and take a very close look at just how much of what you're eating is carbohydrate.

If the general concept of carb-counting is new to you, simply type "carb-counting" into your Internet search engine, and you will have more than a few choices of ways to learn the basics!

Whether you choose to eat a low-carb diet or a high-carb diet, or somewhere in between, awareness about carbohydrates is vital to your life with diabetes, and for most people, it will be the key to success in their weight-loss and blood sugar goals. Then what? Well, with the support of your doctor, it may be beneficial to try reducing your carbohydrate intake, gradually, by substituting some of your carb-packed choices with more whole food proteins and veggies.

8. Experiment with Removing Gluten and/or Dairy from Your Diet for Three Weeks

These two food groups are the most likely to cause inflammation, irritation, and a variety of negative consequences throughout your entire body. You *do not* have to test positive for celiac disease or lactose intolerance in order to be experiencing negative effects from either of these food groups. They are infamous for symptoms ranging from depression, acne and rashes, inability to lose weight, infertility, fatigue, headaches, joint pain, gas, constipation, and overall vitamin depletion.

Approach the nutritional changes with grace and patience and commitment. Remove the stress of "trying to find something to eat" by seizing the opportunity of learning how to feed your body with different foods than you're used to.

For example, on the gluten-free lifestyle, people often say to me, "There's nothing to eat!" but I'm here to tell you there is *a lot* to eat that is gluten-free without even stepping into the gluten-free baked-goods isle. *Real* food is naturally gluten-free (and a large percentage of processed food is packed with gluten). Remember, removing gluten doesn't necessarily mean you have to go buy a dozen gluten-free alternatives that are incredibly dense in carbohydrates—instead, find your way to the *real whole foods*.

Take a deep breath and research and learn and have fun while you're at it! The proof is in the pudding: if you feel better after those three weeks and then reintroduce gluten and/or dairy into your diet again, you will realize just how much those food groups were impacting your body.

9. Get Rid of Your Scale, Right Now

If your only motivation for improving how you eat is based on your weight and the number on the scale, then your focus is on the wrong thing. Literally, remove the scale from your house and stop obsessing about that number. Your weight is just one of the *many* measurements that can be used to assess your health. Not to mention that healthy weight-loss actually happens *really* slowly. The weight-loss you experience from your nutritional improvements often might not show up on the scale until a couple of months have passed! If you're too focused on the scale, you'll likely quit and give up before you've even gotten to see those results.

When I was at my most fit, most conditioned, most athletic level of training, I weighed 15 pounds *more* than I weigh right now! More! The number on the scale is just one aspect of your health. Sure, at a certain point, using a scale to assess how things are going can be helpful, especially when you've reached your goal weight and you're aiming to maintain that weight, but when you're really at the start of your weight-loss efforts, you don't need that feisty gadget!

Get rid of that scale! Seriously. Right now. Instead, find motivation and take pride in how you feel when you take the time to make yourself a really great dinner of whole foods, or take a photo of your grocery cart when it's packed with 90 percent fresh foods rather than boxes of processed junk. Keep your attention on the tiny details that lead to eventual weight-loss.

10. Focus on YOU and You Alone

In life with diabetes, it's easy to feel like everyone around you can "eat whatever they want" and fill their faces with gross food without any consequences. This type of envious resentment leads to one thing: self-pity. And self-pity leads to simply rebelling against your diabetes by eating food in a way that purposefully harms your health. The reality is that *everyone* is affected by the way they feed their bodies, but some of those people won't see the consequences as quickly as we might because we live with diabetes.

Literally, *everyone* is affected by the way they feed their bodies. The next time you find yourself feeling jealous or angry at the sight of a really fit-looking-person, remind yourself of two things: (1) That person probably puts a lot of energy every day into looking so fit by making great choices about food and exercise, and (2) that person may have one day struggled with her weight just like you might be now, but applied an immense amount of energy, discipline, and patience to get where she is today.

Focus on *your* body. Your well-being. Your health. Your nutritional needs and the awesome benefits that *you* will gain each time you make a great choice about food.

Creating Goals about Food in Life with Diabetes

In Chapter 3, we talked about creating realistic, achievable … *awesome goals* for any part of your life with diabetes. To give you a running start, here are a few examples of small but powerful changes related to food that you can focus on making in your life:

I'm going to:

- *make one meal a day that consists completely of whole, clean foods for the next month.*
- *learn how to prepare and cook one new healthy recipe each week for two months.*
- *eat gluten-free Mondays thru Thursdays for the next three weeks.*
- *replace my late-night binge eating with healthy foods instead of junk foods for one week.*
- *write down why I am eating every time I want to binge on food for one month.*
- *commit to treating low blood sugars with only ___ grams of carbohydrates for two weeks.*
- *prepare chicken on Sundays for the entire week's lunch meals for one month.*
- *treat myself to one dessert every other day for the next three weeks.*
- *simply write down how I feel, emotionally and physically, after every meal I eat for two weeks.*

With the six-step process outlined below, think about the first goal you'd like to create around your life with food today.

1. **Understand where you're starting from**
2. **Be super, extremely, incredibly specific**
3. **Make sure you can measure your progress**
4. **Ask yourself *why* this matters to you**
5. **Establish the tiny, supportive details**
6. **Create a Pick-Up Plan**

_____

_____

_____

_____

_____

_____

_____

_____

_____

_____

_____

_____

_____

_____

_____

_____

———————————————————————————————

———————————————————————————————

———————————————————————————————

———————————————————————————————

The phrase "to each their own" couldn't apply more when talking about the quirky habits and behaviors or not-so-helpful coping methods we each develop about food. The following are anonymous statements collected through a survey on how living with diabetes has impacted or changed the way some people think about or behave around food.

How Diabetes Has Changed the Way I Think and Act around Food...

"Now I actually think about food. I've eliminated (or cut way back) on foods I loved for 60 years, like those comforting bowls of Raisin Bran cereal with really cold milk late at night. I eat less and less ice cream, another 60-year addiction. I'm far from perfect, but now I always at least consider the consequences of what I'm putting inside me. I'm thinking about food consequences always, even when I choose to have that momentary, conscious slip-up. I live with my condition on my mind through both my successes and my failures."

"When my daughter was diagnosed, I remember the doctor telling me 'It's not your fault. You didn't give her diabetes because you fed her one too many happy meals.' I swear he must have read my thoughts. She had an evening dance class on Tuesdays and Thursdays. It was convenient to drop by on those days and pick up a happy meal ... so I still felt responsible and the child has not had a happy meal since. She is still a child, so she does enjoy birthday cake and treats at school. At home we cut out the prepackaged meals and replaced them with fresh

---

(continued)

(*continued*)

How Diabetes Has Changed the Way I Think and Act around Food...

vegetables and fruits. It was hard at first but health overrules conveni-ence. The change benefitted us all."

❧

"Now I think about the nutritional content of everything I eat. I used to eat mindlessly. Now I must stop and think before I put any-thing in my mouth. I have become much more aware of how different foods affect my blood sugar. I always have blood sugar treatments with me and before I exercise I must consider my carbs and insulin and adjust accordingly."

❧

"I was young when I was diagnosed, so all meals were being pre-pared for me. Now I'm an adult and responsible for feeding myself. I try to be conscious of nutrient intake, and whether or not I'm fueling myself well for a healthy life. When faced with a tempting dessert or high-carb food, I think carefully about whether it's worth the effort of complex carb-counting (and potential blood sugar fallout!). I've stopped going on nighttime binges, which I did occasionally in my teens and early twenties (before and after diagnosis). One challenge I'm working on now is fitting in time to cook healthy meals amid my busy schedule. I recognize how important it is, but still have a habit of going for convenient foods!"

❧

"I eat a lot healthier. I eat way more fruits and veggies now. I also read labels. I never used to read labels."

❧

"Being a diabetic has made me much more aware of how diges-tion and metabolism works. I eat in ways that would be healthy for anyone, diabetic or not. I was pretty young when I was diagnosed (age 12) so I wasn't very deliberate about my eating before diagnosis. However, I had poor glucose control for the first 15 years of diabetes.

(*continued*)

(continued)

How Diabetes Has Changed the Way I Think and Act around Food...

Once I figured out how to eat limited amounts of fast-acting carbs and use less insulin, things got much better."

❧

"I learned how to count carbs. I learned (from a TeamWild's online training program) the benefits of carbs and why I need them for fuel during endurance exercise. I started using a pump which helps me to feel more relaxed about eating when I want to. I also use the My Fitness Pal app to look up carb-counts, keep track of what I am eating, and collect data on my intake (including fats, proteins, carbs, etc.). Recently I have cut down on processed carbohydrates and am noticing the difference in my blood sugars. I try to get regular exercise to support my metabolism, burn calories, and decrease stress. When I am exercising regularly I make better food choices."

❧

"I build 'things' with food. I now use toothpicks, drink umbrellas, and all kinds of fun accessories to make the 'good' foods enjoyable for kids. One day when I asked my son what he wanted for lunch ... his response was 'a plateful of disappointment, 'cause that's all that's in the fridge.' So, I had to get creative. I made a big smiley face out of fruit and toothpicks. Thus began my food-art."

❧

"I used to binge—nothing extreme like an entire pack of Oreos in one sitting, but I would feel hungry or bored or crave a particular thing and then eat a whole string of snacks in a row. This habit fell away over time without much conscious effort, but two things helped. One, I started filling up my schedule with fun stuff that didn't focus on food—that way I would distract myself from any negative feelings that caused me to eat. Two, I reminded myself of the consequences of bingeing. Invariably, I would wake up in the morning with a high blood sugar, feeling sluggish and guilty for eating so much the night before. After a while, I would get a craving and think, 'Is it worth the bad feelings afterwards? I'd rather

(continued)

(continued)

How Diabetes Has Changed the Way I Think and Act around Food...

feel good.' Sometimes binges resulted from a low blood sugar and the panic-eating that followed. One thing that has helped with that is exercise. Regular, intense exercise helps my body to create glycogen more easily, which means my lows have become less severe. This helps me maintain a sense of calm and control when my brain is blitzing out on hypoglycemia, which therefore leads to self-restraint on treating lows. Intense exercise is key, though—you have to push!"

∾

"I don't skip breakfast anymore. I also tend to eat the same amount but I spread it out into smaller meals instead of eating three bigger meals each day."

∾

"I started small. I used to eat white bread only—so I started with one change a month. First month was brown bread, then it was brown rice, brown pasta, adding more vegetables, planning one meatless dinner a week. I can't change everything all at once, so I do little bits at a time. Better results!"

∾

"I escaped the cycle of carb cravings by limiting starches and fast-acting carbohydrates. Once they didn't seem to be a necessity I had a healthier relationship with them. I use starches in my diet like seasoning, a taste here and there, and very little impact on my blood sugars."

∾

"Serving size considerations—I follow them more!"

∾

"When I was first diagnosed four years ago, I thought, 'No problem, I will just keep my blood sugar between 70 and 120.' Ha, was I ever in for a surprise! Being diagnosed with diabetes motivated me to work hard to take care of myself in order to live a long healthy life without complications. At least without complications related to diabetes!"

(continued)

(*continued*)

How Diabetes Has Changed the Way I Think and Act around Food...

"I realized what effect a lot of foods have on the blood glucose level and overall mood of a smaller child with type 1 diabetes. So, I figured food affects everyone! Family food makeover time!"

"I realized that I often felt bad after eating poorly. I was tired, had stomachaches, experienced crazy blood sugars, and would beat myself up for making those choices. When I eat well, I feel good! When I eat something that I know the exact carb-count for, I feel in control. And the sense of being in control really helps when I'm burned-out with diabetes. I also am motivated by the future. I want to live a long and healthy life with diabetes. Making smart food choices and eating a healthy diet are cornerstones to that goal. Keeping that long-term vision in mind helps in the day-to-day grind of deciding what to eat."

"I've seen how family members with diabetes struggled when they didn't change their nutritional habits and I didn't want to be like them. I learned from their bad examples."

"I was denied life insurance at age 30. I was determined to win, so I fixated on getting a stellar A1C and got it. It took me about six months to sort out my blood work and qualify for life insurance. Since then, I've been motivated to have as close to normal blood sugars all the time. I never feel guilty or imbalanced about it. It's just part of who I am, and I do my best, with a few slips here and there."

"I was gaining weight, felt terrible, felt weak, my bones hurt, my joints hurt. I hated looking in the mirror. And I felt like a failure in my diabetes and in my life. I am getting older and my food needs are changing and I needed to address that. I feel better when I eat better, I sleep better and my 'in range' blood sugars are proof that eating well is a good choice!"

Rome Wasn't Built in a Day

Remember, nothing has to change *tomorrow* and, in the bigger picture, this is a long-term process of simply learning more about the food, how you feel when you eat different types of food, and a gradual process of appreciating how good you feel when you eat one thing and how not-so-good you feel when you eat something else. It's a natural process that many of us have gone through, in our own way, but it starts with *wanting* a change in your life, in your diabetes, in your relationship with food.

And now, let's hope you didn't just finish a big meal, because we're gonna talk about exercise!

Get Your Sweat-Betes On!

6

Learning How to Make Exercise of Any Kind a Real (and Positive!) Part of Your Life

If you live with diabetes, then you can officially call any form of exercise or activity you engage in "sweat-betes." Mostly, because it's funny to say … and that's really the only reason. (I didn't make up the term, and I honestly don't know who did!) But it doesn't change the fact that there are five things that make regular sweat-betes challenging:

1. **Attitude:** The way you think about exercise and the things you tell yourself about exercise will absolutely determine whether or not it becomes a real part of your life.
2. **Making the time:** Whether or not you have diabetes, making the time to exercise in your busy life isn't always easy, and it can require some prioritizing and shifting in how you use your day.
3. **Getting started:** If you're someone who currently doesn't exercise at all, knowing how to get started and what kind of exercise you should even start doing can be really overwhelming.
4. **Balancing your blood sugars:** If you take insulin, and especially if you live with type 1 or type 1.5 diabetes, the biggest challenge about exercise comes down to keeping your blood sugar from dropping too low or rising too high.
5. **Pressure. Pressure. Pressure:** Whether the pressure comes from magazines, their doctor, their mom, or their youngest child, there is inevitable pressure on people with diabetes to exercise every day. And that pressure, just like the pressure about food, can backfire big time.

In the end, though, the reason there's a chapter on *exercise* in a book about diabetes burnout is because exercise is truly a powerful tool for living happily with diabetes—not just because it's "good for your blood sugar," like your doctor says, but because it's good for your soul, your spirit, your mind. And yes, in a way, the *pressure* to exercise can add to the burnout, but we're gonna talk about that and make sure it doesn't get in the way of your ability to get active.

All five of the things on that list above matter, and all five need attention in order for you to make sweat-betes a real part of your life. I'm sure what you *don't need* is to hear about more research studies proving the benefits of exercise on blood sugars and life with diabetes. We hear and read about those every day, in every newspaper and website. But if you're struggling with your blood sugars and struggling with your energy and your mood and stress, and you *aren't* exercising, then you're missing one of the key ingredients that will lessen those struggles.

In the spring of 2012, I had to stop lifting weights because of a mysterious pain in several areas of my body that seemed to have no clear diagnosis. Throughout the following two years, I tried every type of exercise I could think of to find one that didn't hurt me as I continued to experience pain in more areas of my body, including my ankles, feet, wrists, elbows, neck, and knees. For about six months, I did almost zero exercise other than casual walks in the woods with my dogs while being tested for multiple sclerosis, Lyme disease, brain tumors, injuries, nerve damage, rheumatoid arthritis, and a variety of weird and rare conditions I can't even remember.

After just the first six months of being so inactive, I gradually felt less and less like myself. Suddenly I wondered, "Why am I so unhappy? I don't have any legitimate excuse to be *this* unhappy and down … what's going on? And man alive, why am I so *tired?*"

The *only* change I had made was my activity level. My nutrition was great. I was actually losing weight because I wasn't powerlifting anymore and my appetite had dropped significantly as a result. My blood sugars were fine. But my body *and mind* were desperately out of whack simply because I wasn't exercising.

By 2014, I was finally diagnosed with fibromyalgia after a clear month-long flare-up. Fibromyalgia is a condition characterized by inconsistent widespread pain, trouble sleeping, fatigue, and depression.

Today, I'm wholeheartedly committed to walking several miles every day. Some days are more painful than others. I wear a specific brand of tennis shoes (I've never played tennis) that keep the pain in my feet and knees at a minimum when I'm walking. Even though I can't feel that same awesome pump of blood through my muscles as after an intense powerlifting workout, I feel like myself again simply from the low-impact exercise of walking. Also, making that active, conscience decision to do something good for myself, to spend an hour or two of my day doing something *really* good has intangible rewards to my self-esteem and overall self-respect.

I could go on and on about the benefits of exercise, but it will only matter to you when you truly feel them for yourself. They are real. The benefits can impact every part of who you are, including your self-esteem. You deserve to exercise your body. You are worth it.

You may have obstacles—believe me, I get it—but finding *something* that works for you is not just important for your blood sugars, it's also important for your spirit and your mind.

So, let's take a closer look at five areas that need your utmost attention when working to make exercise a bigger part of your life:

1. Make It a Priority, Baby!

"I don't have time." I hear this a lot, but all I really want to ask in response to this is, "How many hours of TV do you watch each day?" Sure, it's possible that some people really have crazy, busy schedules, but for most of us, there is at least 30 minutes we could create for ourselves by getting out of bed 30 minutes earlier or spending 30 minutes less watching TV every day. Roll out of bed and go for a walk—you don't even have to get in your car!

Getting out of bed 30 minutes earlier (with an alarm clock, or even more than one, that force you out of bed to turn them off) *or* ensuring that the moment you get out of work you can easily pop into your gym clothes and head to the gym are decisions that only you, and you alone, can make.

If you want to let the excuse that you "don't have time to exercise" rule your life, that's your choice, but I guarantee there are some very busy people in the world who still make exercise a major priority. Whether it means recording your favorite TV show for later, getting a friend to meet you at the gym or a yoga class, or simply deciding that the 30 minutes you spend vegged out on the couch each night could be 30 minutes you actually spend at the gym ... pick a time of day, and make it happen!

2. It Doesn't Have to Be Every Single Day!

Sure, exercising every day would be awesome, but if you're working on making this a bigger priority, don't over-commit and find yourself burned out barely two weeks into your new regimen.

If you *really* haven't been exercising at all lately, then pick just two or three days of the week that you will commit to exercising. And guess what? It *doesn't* have to be for 60 minutes or more in order to count. If your 30 minutes of strength-training are serious and intense, that's awesome, and that's plenty!

In fact, maybe you could even start with a goal of just *one* day of exercise per week. For example, "Today, I'm going to go for a walk." Take away the expectation of having to do it again and again and again, and just create a goal for that very one day. Give yourself the chance to enjoy the time you spend walking. Think of it as *your* time.

After several years of training for two hours every day, I have found awesome joy out of giving just 30 minutes of energy to intense bodyweight strength-training (plus a variety of dog walks), and have had awesome results. Neither way is necessarily wrong or right—they each have different goals and purposes. But both are great. Ease in gradually based on your personal level of fitness.

3. Learn More so You Don't Waste Your Time!

Wasting your time in the gym is a really easy thing to do if you haven't taken the time to educate yourself about good-quality exercise. You don't need to research very deeply in order to learn that jogging for 30 minutes every day is actually *not* the best way to lose weight, or to learn that weightlifting with 5- to 8-pound dumbbells for 50 or more reps, is also not a very effective way to build any strength! The knowledge is out there, but you have to go seek it!

Quality is much more important than quantity.

Two suggestions to maximize your time at the gym:

1. Try using dumbbells that are heavy enough for you to hit "failure" after 12 to 15 repetitions. Don't be afraid to increase the weight when it's appropriate.
2. Instead of jogging at the same pace (which burns far more glucose than fat), try doing intervals of sprinting (whatever a "sprint" is for your level of fitness) on a treadmill or any cardio equipment for 60 seconds, followed by 60 seconds of walking for 20 to 30 minutes. If 60 seconds feels too long or too short, adjust the time as you need to in order to fit your fitness level, but do not cross the two-minute threshold, especially for your sprinting interval, because that will cause you to start burning more glucose than body fat.

4. Getting Started

You need to try new things in order to find the right type of exercise for your mind and your body! I recently even tried a dance class called "Nia dancing" which I *never* expected to like (because I'm a horrible dancer), but it turned out to be really fun and different. Meanwhile, I tried a tai-chi class and was surprised that I really didn't like it at all.

Consider making a list of a variety of exercises you've never tried and commit to trying each one at least once.

Remember, everybody has to start somewhere. Get over your fears of being the new person in the class or looking foolish—everybody was a newbie at some point. I can guarantee that most people in the gym or a fitness class are far more worried about how *they* look and far less concerned with what you're doing. (We're a self-absorbed species, what can I say?) So leave your inhibitions at the door and just focus on the experience. And hey, a great way to feel more comfortable is to bring a friend along with you!

5. *Balancing Your Blood Sugars*

"My blood sugar always drops too low or goes too high." *This* is a legitimate frustration, but it's not an excuse. If it was impossible to keep our blood sugar in range more often, then there wouldn't be a single famous athlete with diabetes, but there are plenty of such incredible role models! The only difference between such athletes and the person who might give this excuse is that the athletes took the time to learn what their bodies needed during different types of exercise. They saw every blood sugar as information, not a reason to give up.

But managing blood sugars during exercise is not an easy or quick little conversation. Let's dig into some real and useful tips and knowledge for balancing your sweat-betes balancing act.

The Lows and Highs of Exercise and Blood Sugars

You can't read a newspaper or meet with a doctor without being told how important exercise is in life with diabetes, but what many newspapers and medical experts seem to forget is that for people taking insulin, balancing your blood sugar during exercise can be incredibly frustrating! And that frustration just might lead you to give up on exercise, or at least to dread it.

There is no doubt that exercising with diabetes is about one million times more challenging than exercising without diabetes, particularly if you take insulin. Low blood sugars and high blood sugars are major party-poopers in the middle of a walk, yoga, spinning class, tai chi, strength-training … you name it! I'm here to tell you that *it can be done* and you *can enjoy exercise*. But it takes a little work, a little more effort, and a bunch of self-study.

What I really hope, though, is that if you find yourself often angry about your blood sugar during exercise, take a step back and look at this situation with an entirely new perspective. The truth is that your blood sugar is *not* actually doing random, inexplicable, illogical things during exercise. The truth is that there is a physiological process and there are basic variables that determine what types of exercise raise or lower blood sugar. They're normal, they're documented, and maybe you just haven't had a chance to learn about that process and those variables. (And believe me, you totally *can learn* it!)

When I personally started to become really active and committed to exercising regularly, I was working *really* hard to balance my blood sugar during things like Ashtanga yoga, strength-training, and various forms of cardio like power-walking and the Stairmaster. And it wasn't easy, but at the very same time I was learning with the help of my trainer, Andrew, about what was literally going on in my body during different types of exercise. Learning about this basic science, taking a deep breath, and viewing my body as a science experiment is the only reason I am able to exercise happily and confidently today. (And believe me, the moment I try a new type of exercise, I have to recreate that science experiment.)

No stress. No anger. No resentment. Just patience. Openness to learn. And determination!

Top Five Tips for Balancing Blood Sugars during Exercise

1. Understand What Type of Exercise You're Doing

Jogging and strength-training will both have very different impacts on your blood sugar, even though your heart rate may rise during both. Cardiovascular or aerobic exercise uses glucose primarily for fuel. This means that jogging, running, the elliptical, power-walking, cycling, power yoga, and even gardening—anything that raises your heart rate for an extended period of time—will lower your blood sugar.

Anaerobic activity, like strength-training, sprinting, interval, or circuit training—during which your heart rate goes up, then down, up, then down, and muscle is being broken down—is going to burn more fat for fuel during the activity, but may increase your sensitivity to insulin later in the day while it works to repair and build those muscles. It's also very common to see your blood sugar *rise* during this type of exercise, and it's totally normal (and actually promotes strength-gains, etc.)! More mellow forms of exercise, like casual walking or gentle yoga, aren't likely to raise your heart rate high enough to actually burn glucose, but that depends on the individual.

2. Control as Many Variables as Possible

When you're starting a new form of exercise and want to know how that work-out is going to impact your body on a regular day with a "regular" blood sugar, be sure to eat a meal you already know the carbohydrate count of, and don't start your workout with an out-of-range blood sugar (over 180, under 80).

For example, when I switched from powerlifting in the afternoons to doing bodyweight-only plyometric training first thing in the morning (back when I was still trying to find intense forms of exercise I could do without pain), I set up every workout in the beginning to be as similar as possible so I didn't have variables like food or high blood sugars (which can require different correction doses before exercise compared to a nonexercising part of the day), and I performed my workout at the same time of day.

I quickly learned that when I wake up first thing in the morning, with an in-range blood sugar, I can perform my bodyweight workout on an empty stomach and I need one unit of insulin to actually keep my blood sugar from rising. For me, this is the ideal time for exercising because my energy is at its highest and I like to get my workout taken care of before I get started with the rest of my day. However, after confirming this experiment, I also tested what happens if I perform this same type of exercise in the afternoon and my insulin needs are exactly the same. That does *not* mean this applies to *all forms* of exercise. Just this one. If I want to go swimming in the middle of the afternoon, I'll create a new experiment and anticipate different results.

3. Treat Your Low Blood Sugars with Only a Few Types of Foods

The food you choose to treat your low blood sugars with *does* make a differ-ence, not only in the amount of calories you're consuming but also in how quickly your blood sugar will rise. Using a glass of milk or a peanut butter sandwich to treat a low before exercising is going to give you a lot more calories than you really need *and* the fat and protein will slow down the digestion, prolonging when your blood sugar will be safe for exercise again. If you're worried about going low again, use fat and protein *after* treating with a fast-acting carbohydrate to help sustain your blood sugar. (In many cases, though, this really isn't necessary. Low blood sugars just require more patience than we'd like to give them!)

I use juice boxes or juice from a bottle at home. Like I mentioned earlier, I keep Gummy Life Savers in my car because they don't melt or freeze. Juice boxes come with me into the gym, and I keep dried pineapple chunks next to my bed because they are so packed with sugar I only have to eat one or two to bring a low blood sugar back up in the middle of the night. *(I have fallen asleep after realizing I'm low due to literally dreading having to consume another juice box and procrastinating the process! The pineapple goes down much easier for me when I'm half-awake.)*

I can't stress enough that using low blood sugars as an excuse to binge on food is always doomed for a disaster (as mentioned earlier in the section about "Getting Off the Blood Sugar Roller Coaster").

4. Take Really Great Notes!

Pick one form of exercise. Write down the time of day, your pre-exercise blood sugar, anything you just ate, and any insulin you just took. Then write down exactly what kind of exercise you're doing and for how long you're doing it. Check your blood sugar half-way through your exercise, and again at the end of your workout. If your blood sugar is high, then you know you either didn't need to cut back on your insulin dose for the food you ate, or you didn't need the extra boost of glucose you purposefully consumed for your workout, or you actually *need* a little bit of insulin in your body during exercise. If you're low, then you know you can either cut back on your insulin dosing next time (through basal or bolus insulin) or you can consume more carbohydrates *un*covered by insulin.

Aim to perform the exact same experiment again, adjusted based on the information you gained from your first experiment, and keep repeating until you find the right balance!

To give you another example, I know that if I'm going to swim for 30 minutes after eating breakfast or lunch, I need 15 to 20 grams of carbohydrates on board, *uncovered* by insulin, in order to prevent a low blood sugar. To avoid eating unnecessary calories, I time any cardio (glucose-burning) activity for after a normal meal or snack.

Additionally, if you *do* have a high blood sugar before exercising, don't be surprised if you need nearly half as much insulin to correct that high blood sugar, but take good notes in this situation and find out! I know for my own body that a 50 percent correction dose of insulin is all I need if I'm high before most types of exercise.

5. Trying Exercising First Thing in the Morning, on an Empty Stomach

This is a secret trick from the bodybuilding world. Bodybuilders are constantly trying to burn as much body fat as possible without burning up muscle. Thanks to being surrounded by bodybuilders when I first became serious about exercise, I learned based on normal human physiology that exercising first thing in the morning, on an empty stomach, with an in-range blood sugar, is the easiest time of day to keep your blood sugar from dropping because your body is primed to burn fat for fuel instead of glucose. This is because you have been *fasting* all night long, your body's backup stores of glucose have been used for energy while you were sleeping, and so your body uses fat for fuel instead.

For example, if I was going to go for an intense 60-minute walk in the afternoon, it would absolutely lower my blood sugar if I didn't prepare by consuming extra carbohydrates. However, performing that same 60-minute walk first thing in the morning won't lower my blood sugar at all. (Obviously, keep glucose on hand when you first perform this experiment, just in case, especially if your background insulin needs are not finely tuned.)

However, I know that for *my* body, when I perform anaerobic strength-training types of exercise first thing in the morning (or in the afternoon, for that matter), I need one unit of insulin on board to prevent me from spiking. It's just science. That's all. Take the time to learn and experiment, remembering that an unexpected high or low can simply mean there's something about exercise and the human body that you haven't learned quite yet! With this attitude, diabetes will never stop you from making exercise a regular part of your life.

What's Your Attitude Got to Do with It?

There are two types of perspectives a person can carry with them during exercise: a chore or an opportunity.

As a Chore:

This person shows up and begrudges every moment. When they feel their muscles start to burn—a normal part of strength-training, for example—they quit. When their heart rate starts to increase—a natural reaction to aerobic exercise, for example—they slow down. When they start to get tired, they stop. When they're presented with something new, something they've never done before, they don't even try. Everything seems like life or death, "If I have to do one more round of that exercise, I'll die!" or "I don't think I can do that exercise! I definitely can't!" only to find out in a few moments that they certainly can. This type of exerciser isn't present, mentally, when they're exercising. They show up and do the bare minimum, wishing the whole time that they were somewhere else.

They fear trying something new and allow the fear of failing or struggling to stop them in their tracks. They judge themselves and their abilities constantly rather than focusing on what they are capable of and what they are working toward.

The result? Well, they're putting more energy into resenting their workout rather than putting energy into making the most of their workout … so their results and progress from their exercise reflects that! Wasted time. And it wouldn't be surprising to see this person drop exercise from their daily routine altogether simply because their attitude prevents them from appreciating and enjoying it.

As an Opportunity:

The second kind of person I encounter is a person who sees their daily exercise routine as an opportunity.

This person shows up. And I don't just mean physically, but *mentally*. They know they have the next 45 to 60 minutes to spend on exercise and after that, they'll go back to the rest of their life whether it's sitting in front of a computer or standing behind a counter, or whatever. But for the next hour they are simply *here* to think about exercising their body. They embrace the work. They embrace trying new things and the nervousness of not knowing how difficult or easy it might be. When faced with something new, they say, "I don't know if I can … but I'll try my best and find out!"

This person embraces the challenges of physical movement with a perspective of seeing just what their body is capable of without judgment! This person embraces the feeling of doing something good for herself, embraces the discipline required to show up, and is never afraid to try something new or difficult.

When asked to do more of an exercise, they don't argue or plead that they can't; they simply try to do as much as they safely can. When faced with the choices of staying home on the couch because they're tired or going to the gym because they're tired, they remind themselves that they always feel better after a little exercise. And they see exercise as something that impacts their entire life in a truly positive way.

There's no way to sugarcoat this one: making exercise a bigger part of your life always comes down to a choice. Just like many other aspects of health. Whether you go to a group fitness class, hire a trainer, workout on your own, go for walks or bike rides in your neighborhood, join a yoga studio, attend dance or tai chi classes, or make use of the zillions of free exercise videos on YouTube, it comes down to a choice.

Excuses, Excuses, and Excuses … Oh My!

Excuses are the worst. I put off painting my bedroom, the last bedroom left in our new house to paint, because I had convinced myself I couldn't possibly reach the ceiling with the ladder we owned and my less-than-awesome skills with one of those extendable paint-rollers. (I was pretty sure I'd fall off the ladder and kill myself in a freak painting accident.) And then I got over myself and just *tried*. I said, "Ya know, I might as well give it a try, and if it goes horribly, then I'll just have to suck it up and hire someone."

I could at least *try*. And finally did. And I lived. (And the room looks *so* nice!)

Excuses are dangerous. They can keep us from realizing our true potential. Keep us from becoming the people we want to be. They keep us from trying, simply stepping one foot in front of the other and trying.

Excuses get created in our minds based on all kinds of things like fear, stubbornness, insecurities, resentment, apathy, laziness, and simply a lack of *wanting* something more than the desire you have to keep that excuse alive. Some excuses are ridiculous, such as "I don't like being sweaty," and the personal trainer in me would ask you, "Really? That's worth keeping you from exercise?" And some are really logical, such as if you currently have a medical condition that makes many types of exercise dangerous for you or if you have aches and pains in your body that seem to be exacerbated by exercise.

Of course, many of us have aches and pains and injuries and medical limitations, but there is almost always still some form of exercise you can do to keep your body moving. Almost always. As I mentioned earlier, I personally experience a great deal of discomfort and pain almost every day. It took me a while to feel okay and truly accept the new limits of what I can and cannot do with my body because of that pain. And that wasn't an easy thing to come to terms with for someone who used to compete in powerlifting and teach seven power-yoga classes every week!

But I also know that everything about my body feels better when I do exercise. To me, there's a big difference between doing something that will make an injury worse, and doing something that can cause discomfort but not actually increase or worsen that discomfort. Doing *nothing* just isn't a long-term option in my mind.

We can't let aches and pains keep us on the couch, which is guaranteed to simply cause more aches and pains. Yes, we do *need* to talk to our doctors about our limitations and capabilities, and then find a form of exercise that fits well within those parameters.

Top Three Excuses and Ginger's No-Nonsense Trainer-Like Response!

1. **"I can't afford a gym membership."** If spending money on exercising isn't in your budget, then grab your sneakers and hit the pavement of your neighborhood (getting a friend to be your walking-buddy is awesome, by the way) or search through YouTube for an endless source of videos on practically every kind of exercise you could think of … without spending a penny.
2. **"I don't like being sweaty."** This isn't an excuse, this is just silly. I bet ya don't mind *other* recreational activities that lead to sweatiness, eh? That's all I'm gonna say on that.
3. **"I am too tired."** I'm sure you are, because you haven't made exercise a priority in your life. I could say this a million times but it won't mean anything to you until you experience it for yourself: exercising at the right intensity for you will give you *more* energy.

So now it's time to write down *your* list of excuses that have kept you from exercising, trying something new, or challenging yourself further in exercise:

_____

_____

_____

_____

_____

_____

_____

_____

_____

Now take that list and ask yourself if any of those reasons are truly worth missing out on one of the best ingredients for living a better life with diabetes—or simply a better life regardless of diabetes!

Letting go of these excuses could be as simple as acknowledging that they truly are just excuses, not legitimate reasons for avoiding exercise.

The Pressure to Exercise (Like the Perfect Diabetic)

Yes, there is endless pressure for those of us with diabetes to exercise more, but in reality, there's pressure on *everyone* to exercise more. Even people *without* diabetes are constantly being threatened, "If you don't exercise, you'll develop diabetes!" None of us can avoid it, and for good reason: we *all* benefit from regular exercise.

We can't really make it go away, but we *can* ignore it. Any long-term success you have in exercise will *not* be the result of a person or magazine who pressured you to exercise, but instead because *you* made the choice to exercise.

One way for dealing with those pressures? Explain what kind of support you do or don't need to your friends and family. While we'll talk more about our loved ones in the next chapter, sometimes your significant other might think he or she is being helpful by constantly saying something like, "Make sure you exercise today!" Some people find that really supportive and helpful, while others find it to be an irritating pressure and expectation. If you're someone who doesn't like that form of "support," explain to your loved one that it doesn't make you feel good and tell them what *would* be helpful to you, for example, not mentioning it, being an exercise buddy, or watching the kids so you can have an hour to exercise.

Forget about those orders and demands that you ought to exercise more. Instead, ask yourself if you want to make exercise a bigger part of your life … and *choose* it for yourself. It is your choice. No one else's.

Push those "perfect diabetic" pressures aside and focus on what you want for your own health. You never know, once you remove the negative pressure and thoughts in your head, you may just realize that it feels good to get your heart pumping with a little sweat-betes sometimes!

Remember, you can *choose* to make exercise part of your life and seize the opportunity … or you can resent it altogether. I encourage you to choose your health.

Creating Goals for Exercising in Life with Diabetes

In Chapter 3, we talked about creating realistic, achievable … *awesome goals* for any part of your life with diabetes. To give you a running start, here are a few examples of small but powerful changes you can focus on making in your life around exercise.

I'm going to:

- *wake up 30 minutes earlier to go for a 20-minute walk every other day for one month.*
- *go for a walk with my coworker during my lunch-break Monday thru Thursday for three weeks.*
- *try one new type of fitness class every week for one month.*
- *pick one new exercise video on YouTube to do after work every Monday, Tuesday, and Thursday for the next two months.*
- *push myself a little harder at the gym by increasing my time spent on the treadmill by five minutes every week for three months.*
- *commit to exercising four times each week and checking it off on my calendar for two months.*
- *promise that when I feel "too tired" after work, I will go to the gym for at least 10 minutes before I can go home to rest for the next month.*
- *choose three types of exercise that intimidate me the most and give them all at least one try during the next month.*

With the six-step process outlined below, think about the first goal you'd like to create concerning your life around exercise today.

1. **Understand where you're starting from.**
2. **Be super, extremely, incredibly specific.**
3. **Make sure you can measure your progress.**

4. Ask yourself *why* this matters to you.
5. Establish the tiny, supportive details.
6. Create a Pick-Up Plan.

_____

_____

_____

_____

_____

_____

_____

_____

_____

_____

_____

_____

_____

_____

_____

_____

_____

_____

_____

_____

But You Ain't in This Alone!

Alright, alright, but now we've gotta talk about all those people in your world who care about you! That's right, because whether we like it or not, our friends and our family *want* to be there for us … except, sometimes they don't quite know what the best kind of support looks like. So it's our job to teach them!

What Others Have to Say: On Being an Athlete with Diabetes

Bradford Gildon, amateur elite triathlete, living with type 1 diabetes

With my athletic endeavors, I measure a lot of metrics for training—watts of power on my bicycle training, miles per minute pacing thresholds during my run training, splits for various yardage distances when swim training—plus the extra measurement and analysis of blood glucose before and during exercise; my insulin management (basal and bolus adjustments); the intensity and duration of exercise I'm doing; the time of day of the exercise, etc.

Trying to keep track of all of these can cause burnout. I try to make mental notes of some of these, but if I don't record all of them, I no longer stress about it. Exercise is supposed to be fun! Without keeping this as a primary motivation of why I'm even doing these types of activities, then I also experience burnout.

I eat well, but it is definitely not "perfect" by any means! I am not a coffee drinker, but I do love Diet Coke. I know lots of athletes who will not drink any carbonated beverages whatsoever—I'm not one of them! I set athletic goals for myself, but I also allow myself to have freedoms such as enjoying some ice cream from time to time. Without these allowances, I would definitely be burned out very frequently.

(continued)

(continued)

What Others Have to Say: On Being an Athlete with Diabetes

Diabetes can be hard. Balancing diabetes and intense exercise can be even *harder*. Not every day will be a perfect day. To pursue your goals and achieve them makes the battle completely worthwhile. Finding something *outside of exercise* about which you are passionate can go a long way in helping you when the diabetes management gets complicated or causes issues with workouts or races. I like to work on projects—wood projects around the house, tinkering on my bikes or my motorcycle—to give me some distraction. I am able to focus my energy on something else rather than just letting the dissatisfaction build up inside of me without a way to let it out. These times really help provide me with a "reset" where I can get away from the day's frustration either regarding a difficulty with my diabetes management, or with a difficulty I encountered during a workout.

Catherine Vancak, professional dancer, living with type 1 diabetes
(DanceThruBeetus.blogspot.com)

When I was first diagnosed I was terrified of making a mistake from a high or low blood sugar because of how it would impact my dance training. I would have moments when I would forget the specifics of a piece I was dancing, or lose my balance during a difficult movement. I never wanted to make excuses and say that it was because of the diabetes, but it really was my diabetes getting in the way. Once I was able to admit that my diabetes really was affecting my dancing, I was better able to manage it. Ignoring my diabetes, would only make things more difficult.

I'm a dancer, so I have a type A personality already. I like to have things under control and my diabetes management is no different.

(continued)

(continued)

What Others Have to Say: On Being an Athlete with Diabetes

I write down everything I eat, I have a schedule of training and rehearsals and I do my very best to stick to them. I know for a fact that the healthier I am, the better I can dance. As a dancer, you're very focused. When you have other responsibilities like many of us do, it can take that focus away from your health. What makes it difficult these days is trying to go to school as well as dance. I am getting close to applying to dental school and each grade on my transcript counts. Trying to organize diabetes around dance as well as exams, labs, and lectures is what I struggle with sometimes.

When I'm burned-out, I won't check my blood sugar as often. My pump will alarm for me to check and I'll just look at my DexCom to get a rough estimate. I try to get by on the bare minimum. If I know a half-cup of cereal is around 15 carbs, I'll just bolus for it and not get into the specifics on the label. I'll sometimes stress eat during exams and if I'm burned-out, I won't bolus properly since I'm so stressed I forget how many cookies I ate! Sometimes I can get away with it, and other times it will come back to bite me.

When I'm burned-out, it affects my whole life, not just my dancing. I tend to have more lows in company class and sometimes I've even been reduced to tears. I just get exhausted. I've danced in companies that didn't acknowledge that I was dealing with this difficult disease, and I've danced in others that used my diabetes as the reason for any mistake I made. Luckily, with lots of work and patience I am able to keep my blood sugars steady and this allows my dancing to continue to improve. Knowing that a healthy body improves my athleticism motivates me to manage my diabetes properly, and since my goal is to continue my athleticism, I keep my body healthy. It's a circle.

(continued)

(*continued*)

What Others Have to Say: On Being an Athlete with Diabetes

Most of life is simply showing up, so show up, keep going, and you'll get to the other side. Burnout, while it may seem endless, is only temporary.

Terena Wilkens, avid cyclist, living with type 2 diabetes

I have not always been athletic, but I did bike everywhere when I was in high school. I lived in a small town and to get to anywhere meant going for a 10 to 12 mile ride. I also participated in the Tour of Saints, a local 50-mile bike tour, while in high school and college. I stopped biking when I went to grad-school in West Virginia, where it was much harder to bike due to terrain, traffic, and time.

Before I was diagnosed in August of 2010, I was trying to lose weight, but instead I was completely exhausted after exercising (and for the rest of the day) and I found myself gaining weight! I was eating fairly healthy, so this just made life more frustrating and it was hard to stay motivated.

I started biking after meeting Ginner Ruddy at the American Diabetes Association's Diabetes Expo in Minneapolis. She persuaded my friend to join the Tour de Cure and, I admit, I went along somewhat reluctantly. I agreed to do 7 miles, but ended up doing 27 miles! I am now co-captain of Team RED Twin Cities, and this year, I rode 45 miles.

My work schedule is really one of the hardest parts of my balancing act. I work at a college in the theatre and dance department

(*continued*)

(continued)

What Others Have to Say: On Being an Athlete with Diabetes

working in technical theatre. My schedule includes long days, late nights, and high stress. I have learned to stock up on healthy foods that I can grab on-the-go. The other issue is really the learning curve of finding out what I need to know and how much and how often I have to eat and exercise for maximum health and physical ability.

My biggest diabetes burnout time is winter because in Minnesota it is cold outside, gets dark early, and my motivation is low. I like to have events in the near future to keep me motivated, but in December, those events are too far out. Going to the gym can also be harder as winter is when gyms are the busiest.

I also find motivation to start is not my strong point. I always feel better when I get out on my bike, but getting out there is sometimes hard. I often push myself to do 10 miles: "Just 10 miles! Forget the wind, the humidity and clouds, just do those 10 miles!" I don't think I have ever actually done *just* 10 miles on those days; it always turns out to be more like 28!

I also find it hard to battle the negative image that people have of type 2 diabetics. I have been told I "brought it on myself," and how I should "exercise more and eat less sugar," and that I have "the fat peoples' disease." Sometimes the negative things people say make me want to give up out of frustration. I have had people close to me discourage me from doing an event because, in their words, it would be hard for me. I have learned to turn that around and now use that to battle the burnout and prove to them, and more so to myself, that "YES, I can!"

(continued)

(continued)

What Others Have to Say: On Being an Athlete with Diabetes

Andy Holder, eight-time Ironman Triathlon finisher, living with type 1 diabetes
(InsulinNation.com)

When I was diagnosed with type 1 diabetes at the age of 36, I wasn't a triathlete yet—as a matter of fact, I had never done a triathlon, I didn't own a bike and I didn't know how to swim. So there were a few other things I feared would hold me back athletically; diabetes wasn't atop the list. All kidding aside, I knew I was taking on a lot by striving to finish an Ironman with all the obstacles I had in front of me, but that was exactly why I took on so much—I wanted to do something extraordinary that would inspire and motivate others. That was my main goal. It had nothing to do with winning races or getting medals. Finishing an Ironman in the face of diabetes was a platform, an opportunity, to show people that you can do anything if you have a positive attitude.

Sometimes people around me forget that I have diabetes; they say I make it look so seamless. The irony of making this look seamless and routine is that I am never not thinking about it … and that can wear on you over time. I struggle every day. I struggle to get through workouts without my blood sugar going too low. I struggle to correct a low during a workout, then end up chasing down highs the rest of the day. I struggle during races, when the athletes I am competing with simply have to worry about the hydration, nutrition, and fitness level. All that goes out the window for me if I have a training-induced high blood sugar, or my performance suffers because I'm low. So I do all the things I am supposed to do, I follow the rules, I plan and I prepare, but sometimes, that's not enough, and diabetes takes over.

(continued)

(continued)

What Others Have to Say: On Being an Athlete with Diabetes

When it comes to burnout, in those fleeting moments of feeling sorry for myself, I just wish that I could have a day off. Not a cure, I'll get to the end of the line on that one, but just a day off—of not thinking about it. No testing, no counting carbs, no fiddling with my pump, and no worrying about highs and lows.

Meanwhile, this may sound cavalier, but the only thing we have to work through this is our attitudes. There are too many things with diabetes, in life, that we can't control. So I focus all my energy on my attitude … and usually that gets me to the other side. We have to maintain that positive attitude and try our best to be "on" everyday, but realize this is a marathon and not a sprint. You will have bad days, but if they are outweighed by the good days you're doing okay.

Colette Nelson, CDE and professional female bodybuilder, living with type 1 diabetes
(ColetteNelson.com)

I didn't want to think that type 1 diabetes would stand in the way of my being my best. I remember my doctor telling me when I was diagnosed at age 12 that exercise plays an important role in controlling diabetes. I started working out as a result and thought that it would help make me live longer and be healthier. As I continued training and working out through my adult life, I had a passion for muscle. I didn't think that I would ever be able to get lean enough to compete because when you take insulin you have to deal with treating lows with sugar or carbs. In order to get lean enough to compete you have to follow a strict diet and one that limits carbohydrates.

My last A1C was 6.3%. That was the highest it has been in a few years. Life, different foods, going out for special occasions, dinner

(continued)

(continued)

What Others Have to Say: On Being an Athlete with Diabetes

parties … all make a difference in your diabetes. I never change my attitude toward my management. I test my sugar 10 to 15 times a day and I take insulin injections to match my food and corrections to keep my blood sugar under 120 mg/dL. But, as good as I am about being disciplined—I am not a human pancreas. Insulin is not a cure and is not a perfect science. The body, food, exercise, stress can be unpredictable.

Perfection doesn't exist. I found that the more I was fixated on achieving perfect numbers the more stressed out I became. I had to realize that my diabetes can't always be perfect and now I am able to let it go if I have a blood sugar I am not happy about. The problem with diabetes is it doesn't give you a day off … it is with you 365 days, 24/7. Diabetes is overwhelming if you look at it as *forever* and it is better to just take it day-by-day. I try my best to control my diabetes and not let it control me.

Diabetes burnout is a part of living your life with a disease that never gives you a day off. The key is not letting that feeling make you reckless. I always keep the basics of my diabetes regime as a way of life. Yes, I get upset about always having to test my blood sugar, take all my insulin shots with each meal, and deal with highs and lows … but the reality is if I don't take care of myself, no one else is going to do it for me.

When someone tries to knock me down … I get right back up. That is what diabetes does for someone with athletic ambitions. There is nothing worse than having a low blood sugar while working out in the gym and trying to finish a heavy leg workout. It is frustrating when I am trying to do my cardio after training and I am supposed to do it on an empty stomach but I have to eat because my blood sugar is low.

(continued)

(continued)

What Others Have to Say: On Being an Athlete with Diabetes

The most frustrating is when I start my workout at a perfect blood sugar 90 (5 mmol) and after my workout it goes up to 190 mg/dL. I find a way to get through it. I look at the patterns and figure out why things are happening. I believe there is always a reason why your blood sugars are rising or falling. I look for trends and try experimenting with better ways to achieve the balance I need to be most effective with my training.

Don't let the day-to-day grind of diabetes overwhelm you. Take it one day at a time. Treat each day as its own challenge. In this life we have to surrender control to the universe, but your diabetes is something that you can control. Let your diabetes evolve as you evolve.

Jill Meisen, marathon runner, living with type 2 diabetes
(Hudsuckerproxy.blogspot.com)

I have not always been athletic. Well, I should say, I never considered myself athletic. I played sports, softball, tennis, track and cheerleading, but I was always awkward and built as a sturdy Scandinavian farm woman. My athleticism evolved as a part of my treatment for diabetes.

I never had a weight problem until I turned 25. It was then, of course, that I met my husband, whose family had terrible health issues and habits, and I quickly learned about Steak 'n Shake cheese fries and filet mignon. Prior to that, I was very active, a vegetarian, and never had junk food in our house.

I gained 50 pounds in the first year of our marriage.

(continued)

(*continued*)

What Others Have to Say: On Being an Athlete with Diabetes

I ran in college—not competitively—but for stress release. I only got myself to three miles. When I began to have kids, as close in age as they were, I tried to get out of the house and exercise as much as I could. I've gained and lost the same 80 pounds five times in my life. I lost 50 after having all the kids and began weightlifting—I had a pretty nice body, if I do say so myself, but I could never get a flat stomach back. It was that drive for perfection and stress when I began to go back to work full-time that allowed me to gain it all back again and become a couch potato until I was around 42.

At 42, I went on the HCG diet and lost it all. I successfully kept that off for three years, and I finally, after restarting the C25K program over and over and over again five times, decided I would tackle something on my bucket list: running a half-marathon.

I finished respectably, but I went on to build speed and my personal record is two hours and nine minutes right now, as of December 2012. I ran my first marathon in October 2012 in Chicago, and now I'm 39 pounds *up* from when I first started running. It is a constant battle. And it's not just with weight. Lots of times, I want to sleep in. I want to binge on cookies. I skip workouts. I get pretty resentful of having to keep up the six- to seven-day training regimen so I can just break even.

But diabetes has presented me with the issues of inflammation and hanging on to weight, burning less fat, and metabolizing fuel for energy. My metabolic disorder, I feel, has a part to play in my weight, my mood, my menstrual cycle, and everything that should regulate everything about me. It's difficult to "manage" because you're never "done." It's a constant science experiment, with sometimes not so clear-cut variables that you can manipulate.

(*continued*)

(continued)

What Others Have to Say: On Being an Athlete with Diabetes

Jim Onwiler, avid cyclist, living with type 1 diabetes

I have always had a love of sports and participation in them. In my youth, I played baseball and basketball. As an adult my goals around staying fit were geared toward being a better softball player. When my ball-playing days ended, my fitness suffered. Then about five years ago my niece introduced me to the Tour de Cure (a cycling event organized by the American Diabetes Association) and my passion for cycling has exploded ever since. I rode my first century (that's 100 miles) last August! I continue to ride as often as I can and usually get in over 100 miles per week.

Being diabetic presents several challenges for a cyclist. The biggest is managing my blood sugar. The single most frustrating part of this is having low blood sugar on a ride. Waiting on the side of the road for a number to rise to a safe riding level—*arg!* I always have strategies I've developed in place to manage low and high blood sugars.

We all have days with this disease where things are out of control. For me this usually means blood sugars over 200 that won't come down. Most of the time, in these situations I have learned to understand why I am high and how to get back down. The occasions where I can't explain and can't control find me cursing at my insulin pump, taking correction bolus after correction bolus, and checking my blood sugar every 30 minutes. The hardest part of this ordeal is to not come crashing down too fast only to manage a low.

I try to learn from each of these experiences to understand and better handle them in the future.

(continued)

(continued)

What Others Have to Say: On Being an Athlete with Diabetes

My inspiration to living well with diabetes is life itself. Living a long, happy life to me means staying active.

Cynthia Zuber, avid cyclist, living with type 1 diabetes
(MyDiabetesLight.com)

It was not until living with diabetes for about 20 years that exercise became a key component in my diabetes toolkit. All of the years before I would exercise when the weather was pleasant for Minnesota (we have a long winter …) and maybe a few short-lived stretches throughout the year when I made attempts to work out at a gym with a membership in the fitness facility at my university or apartment complex.

What changed at age 31 for me? I met my husband! He owned an elliptical machine and after we got married, in the dead of winter, I would force myself to make my way down to the basement to exercise on that dang elliptical. I hated it! And it made my foot fall asleep! I would exercise for a few weeks then miss a couple of days that would turn into weeks. During this time I would feel immense shame that would only delay my eventual return to the elliptical.

I finally realized that it did me no good to beat myself up for the days and weeks I missed and to just hop back on. Getting over this self-shaming and punishment piece is what helped me eventually break through and accomplish my goal of making exercise an everyday part of my life. I knew that no one else was going to take

(continued)

(continued)

What Others Have to Say: On Being an Athlete with Diabetes

care of my diabetes and ensure I would be around for a long, healthy and happy life with my husband other than me. It all came down to the effort I put in. I now exercise daily and it is a part of my life just like taking my insulin or testing my blood sugar.

Ryan Attar, CrossFit coach, living with type 1 diabetes

(1HappyDiabetic.com)

Diabetes has inspired me to achieve perfection with my blood sugars. Having healthy blood sugars has really been the inspiration behind me starting my master's degree in nutrition, and now my Naturopathic Physician degree. It started a few years ago, just by reading up on health and nutrition topics, then getting into a great CrossFit gym that had a good nutrition program. Fitness and nutrition really clicked with me, and I then went and got my CrossFit Trainer certification. I then quit my job, and decided to change career paths and started the nutrition degree. So this has been a gradual evolution for me. My next step, becoming a doctor, is a big one, and for sure I'll have many challenges over the next four years.

Blood sugars definitely get elevated during intense CrossFit workouts. I used to bolus before a workout, and this would usually remedy it, but I've found that workouts aren't as predictable as food, so the chance of hypoglycemia is there. I enjoy striving for good numbers.

Crazy Little Thing Called Love 7
This One Is for the People Who Love and Care about You!

Yowza. Having people in your life who love and care about you is *not easy*. I mean, those people actually want to help us and support us and *be there for us* when the going gets rough. Can you imagine? The nerve of these people! Ugh! A nightmare.

Right? Ehhh … maybe not. The rock 'n' roll band Queen wasn't joking when they titled their song, "Crazy Little Thing Called Love." (Oh, believe me, we'll talk about the strangers who don't even know us, let alone love us, and the crazy things that come out of their mouths about diabetes, too.)

You see, the bigger problem is that the words "help" and "support" and "love" are very vague words. To some people, feeling "helped" could feel like total harassment from the diabetes police, and to others, that form of "help" just might not feel like enough!

"Oh, honey, but I love you! That's why I'm always telling you when you're eating too many carbohydrates at breakfast!"

Um … except, it doesn't *feel* supportive. It feels obnoxious and only adds to the guilt we carry on our shoulders every day for not being that perfect diabetic robot. What it means to truly be helpful, supportive, and loving to a person with diabetes can be very confusing, to say the least. And when things get confusing, other emotions like anger and resentment and frustration get going. And those things lead to arguments, yelling, hurt feelings, and in the end *not* a whole lot of love.

I remember a friend of mine in college, who grew up with me and was in school to become a nurse, waving her finger at me like I was a bad,

bad, diabetic after having a bit of dessert at an event. (Yes, she had some dessert, too.)

I remember working as a bartender, having a spoonful of the "damaged" cheesecake that all the waitresses were helping themselves to and seeing the gasp on one colleague's face. "Bad girl!" she teased.

I remember sitting down in a restaurant with my friend and her parents, who proceeded to tell me what I could and couldn't order off the menu because of my diabetes and celiac disease. They truly thought, I'm sure, that they were being helpful, but they left me feeling like my privacy had been invaded, like a sick little child (I was 18 at the time), and simply embarrassed, because no 18-year-old wants to be told how to order food in a restaurant.

But those reminders from our friends and family to check our blood sugar or take our insulin usually come from a good place, right? From a place of wanting to be helpful, supportive, and loving. It's not like we can or even *want* to ask those people to stop caring about us, right? Stop loving us? Stop being there for us? Logically, even though it is not being delivered in the form that we want it to be in, it's a good thing they care so much about us and our life with diabetes, right? And that's one of the hardest things to remember when you're the one living with diabetes and on the receiving end of that love that doesn't feel so helpful.

There are really only two ways to deal with it:

1. Ignore the not-so-helpful love. Get angry about it. Rebel against diabetes because somebody wants you to take better care of yourself. Feel annoyed, confined, pissed off, and claustrophobic because of it. Tell lies so that person will think their help or support or whatever is being received and taken seriously. Cry. Yell. Scream. Roar. You name it.
2. Speak up. Take a deep breath. And communicate to those around you what "help" and "support" and "love" really look like when it comes to your life with diabetes. It's not a fun job. It's not always easy. And hey, it sucks. But if we want the people around us to stop acting like the crazy diabetes police, watching every move we make and every carbohydrate we eat, we need to teach them what really great diabetes help, support, and love looks like.

Not *Enough* Help or Support?

Perhaps the people closest to you don't actually show enough care or concern about your diabetes? While this is probably something that those who feel overly cared for yearn for, you might feel like those closest to you don't actually realize just how much stress and pressure you're under because of diabetes.

Sometimes, this could actually be the way it looks on the outside, but inside those people could be simply intimidated or lacking enough knowledge about what diabetes really is and entails. For others, though, the people who are with you every day, they may be great candidates for a straightforward chat. That chat really would consist of "speaking up" and expressing yourself in many of the same ways a person who feels overly cared for would need to speak up.

Here are a few tips for creating that conversation:

1. Choose a time when everyone is calm, rather than in the midst of a moment when you are frustrated over a high blood sugar and your friend is oblivious, which is only adding to your frustration. In fact, you could even give them a heads-up. "Hey, at dinner tonight I was hoping to talk to you about my diabetes," or "I've been struggling with my diabetes lately, and I was wondering if I could talk to you about a few ways I was hoping you might be able to help me."
2. Express yourself clearly. Give the person you're talking to some very clear examples of what you're struggling with and why it's so challenging. We already know that those who don't have diabetes themselves can't possibly know what a low or high blood sugar feels like, so it's our job to really put that into words, especially since we often don't look as sick on the outside as we actually feel during those fluctuating blood sugars.
3. Give them specific ways of supporting you. The last thing we want to do is leave people feeling as though they are now required to worry about you day and night, right? Instead, give them some very specific examples of what kind of support you'd like to receive from them— just as those who feel overly cared for should do as well. You'll find examples of this later in the chapter.

There are also the people who just totally "get it" right from the start! Like my best friend, Tara, who loves to bake (and run marathons) who has taken the time to understand that I *can* enjoy dessert with a good insulin dose and plenty of blood sugar checks to see how that dose covered the treat. She actually *brings* gluten-free chocolate presents to me every now and then. And during our weeklong vacation (after a powerlifting competition) in Florida, she insisted we hunt for the *best* key lime pie by ordering a slice everywhere we went. (And yes, now I have exceptional skills in the realm of judging key lime pie for the proper tartness-to-sweetness ratio.) And at the very same time, she is one of those people in my life who inspire me to continue taking care of myself, feed myself well, treat myself well, manage my blood sugars well—and she knows that includes some treats now and then.

I also remember growing up with diabetes and having total support from my mom to be imperfect. Literally, in all ways, it was okay. I did the best I could at all times and often, that meant I was imperfect as a kid and a teen living with diabetes.

And I remember every day that I live with my fella, Roger. Every day that passes during which he *doesn't* police my life with diabetes. He gets it. But he gets it because I've been very, very clear about what great support looks like, what kind of support I *do* want from him, and it has to be said: he knows I make great efforts to take care of myself every day, so he doesn't have to worry about the bigger picture of my safety and my life. If I were clearly neglecting my blood sugars, appearing sluggish or sick because of ups and downs and poor eating, he would be worried, and justifiably, he'd step in and speak up. Because he cares about me. And that's a good thing.

On a daily basis, though, he knows how to communicate with me about my diabetes because I've shown and explained to him what I need.

In the end, there's no way we can truly expect those around us to understand what we want for support in life with this disease if we don't take the time to explain it to them. It's a really complicated disease. It can *look* really scary sometimes. It *sounds* scary if someone who loves you has ever read a magazine or watched a story on the news about diabetes. And if we expect the people who love us to just sit back and watch while we struggle or even intentionally neglect our own health life, well, that's kind of crazy. Right? You wouldn't just sit back and *do nothing* if one of your good friends said, "I'm gonna destroy my health really, really gradually over the next few years by doing this, that, and this." Right? Probably not.

There's just no way around it. We've gotta take the time to teach those around us how to behave, speak, and help around our life with diabetes.

And there are *two* categories of people: (1) strangers and acquaintances and (2) our friends and family. First, let's start with the total strangers and acquaintances.

Oh, the Things People (and Total Strangers) Say about Diabetes!

Bill Cosby was wrong, it's not just kids who say the darndest things, it's mature adults and total strangers, too. If you or your child have lived with any type of diabetes for at least five minutes, chances are that someone you know or a complete stranger has said something to you about your diabetes that dropped your jaw to the floor.

That being said, some comments or questions come from a truly curious place, like, "So, are you allowed to eat sugar?" That question isn't offensive, rude, or critical, it's simply a question about life with diabetes. And that's okay, at least for me. I don't mind educating and sharing about my life with diabetes to anyone who is genuinely interested. If I wanted to keep it a secret or not deal with those questions, it would be my responsibility to keep my diabetes management more hidden and not *ever* mention it in casual conversation. It's totally our decision whether we make it public or not, but making it public means we're opening ourselves up to comments and questions.

Sometimes, though, the questions or comments come out with very different intentions or a level of thoughtlessness that leaves you feeling just … ugh.

As a person who is very open about my diabetes (I mean, I can't exactly talk about what I do all day for work without focusing primarily on diabetes and the fact that I live with it), I anticipate and even invite the friendly, well-meaning version of those comments and questions. But every once in a while, there's a question or comment that shocks me. It shocks me because if I were face-to-face with someone living with a chronic illness that I didn't know anything about firsthand, I can't imagine letting such questions or comments come out of my mouth.

I think back to the many times someone has told me they've been diagnosed with any particular kind of cancer, and while I know several people who have actually died due to cancer, the *last* thing I would ever say to that person newly diagnosed is, "Oh, I know someone who died from that." And yet, that response is probably what I've heard *the most often* from friends and strangers in my life with diabetes.

The variety of comments can feel frustrating, hurtful, embarrassing, and infuriating.

Here are my top 29 "favorite" comments and questions spoken to people with diabetes. This list was first published at DiabetesDaily.com.

1. My grandma had diabetes. She lost her leg, then she died. *(Thank you! That's so inspiring!)*
2. You'll die if you eat sugar, right?
3. You have diabetes? You don't look *that* fat. *(Oh ... thanks.)*
4. You take insulin? Oh, you must have the bad kind of diabetes. *(Really? What's the good kind?)*
5. Your *child* has diabetes? Did they get it because you fed them too much candy?
6. Oh my god, you have to take shots every day? I'd die if I had to do that. *(Well, I'd die if I didn't.)*
7. Doesn't that hurt? *(Um, yeah, it's a sharp object going into my body. Duh!)*
8. Well, that sounds better than something like leukemia.
9. Oh my gosh, can you eat that? You can't eat that!
10. That's the disease that causes you to lose your legs, right?
11. I heard you can cure that with diet and exercise. *(Great, that sounds so easy!)*
12. I eat so much sugar, I'm probably gonna give myself diabetes, too!
13. So you just have to avoid sugar, and you're okay, right?
14. Why don't you get a pump that just manages it for you?

15. My friend's daughter has one of those pump things that just manages it for her.

16. Are you allowed to eat that? *(Is it your job to police me?)*

17. You just have to take insulin sometimes, and you're okay, right? *(Yup! It's that simple.)*

18. They say cinnamon can level your blood sugars.

19. They say _____ (any random food) can level your blood sugars.

20. Your kid has diabetes? Well, at least he can grow out of it.

21. You have diabetes and celiac disease? Geeeez, how many diseases do you have?

22. You have diabetes? But you look normal. *(You mean my freaky diabetes features haven't shown yet?)*

23. So you just have to, like, manage it and you're fine? *(Yup, except the "manage it" part is kind of huge!)*

24. You have diabetes? But it seems like you take such good care of yourself?

25. You need to exercise more and you can cure it.

26. You'll die if you have children, right? Like *Steel Magnolias*? *(Nope, thanks a lot, Julia Roberts!)*

27. Ewww! You have to take shots? That is so gross! *(Um, thanks … but it keeps me alive.)*

28. Well, it's your fault, right, for eating too much and not exercising. *(That's incorrect, but also, thanks for your support.)*

29. Oh, you have diabetes? That sucks! *(Yes, thanks for reminding me!)*

There's only so much self-restraint we can apply when someone tells us the chronic illness we live with each day is easily cured by eating more cinnamon. But if we can take a deep breath and respond to some of these comments calmly, we'll help prevent that person from saying the same thing to another diabetic.

Here are a few ways I tackle the three very common and most irritating comments around diabetes. These comments and responses were first published at DiabetesDaily.com.

Comment: *"You'll die if you eat sugar, right?"*

Response: *(Be sure to chuckle a little bit first.) "No, as a person with type 1 diabetes, I have to be very aware of all carbohydrates I eat—whether it's a slice of whole grain bread that your grandmother baked at* *home with the healthiest ingredients in the world, or a handful of Sour Patch Kids. I take a certain amount of insulin every time I eat any type of carbohydrates. In the end, I choose what I eat. My body is just like yours, though: the healthier I eat, the better I feel."*

Comment: "Oh, my grandma had diabetes. She lost her legs and then she died."

Response: (It's okay to grimace a little bit in response to how gruesomely horrifying this comment is.) "Well, back in the day they really didn't have very good technology to check their blood sugars and take their insulin. Today, we have glucose meters that tell us our blood sugars in less than five seconds, and things like insulin pumps and pens that make insulin delivery simpler than having to boil and sharpen the same syringe over and over. These kinds of advances in technology make it possible for people with diabetes to live long, healthy lives."

Comment: "Why don't you just cure your diabetes with weight loss and not eat sugar?"

Response: "Well, first of all you can't cure diabetes—even type 2. I have type 1 diabetes, which means it's completely unrelated to my weight. Type 1 diabetes is autoimmune which means my immune system is attacking the part of my pancreas that makes insulin. That being said, type 2 diabetes is not caused by being overweight or obese, but there is a correlation. Your weight is definitely a contributing factor, and some researchers are trying to determine if it's kind of like the chicken or the egg: which came first? Being insulin-resistant, and having diabetes, can actually cause a person to gain weight long before he or she is diagnosed. Type 2 diabetes is never cured; in many cases it can be managed by things like exercise, healthier eating, and weight loss, but that person will always be diabetic, working hard to manage their blood sugars."

It isn't easy to stay cool and collected in the face of ignorant or hurtful diabetes comments, but if we want to keep such comments from coming over and over, we've gotta make an effort.

Okay, but what about those people who already know the basics of diabetes? I'm talking about the people who really know us, who live with us, who see us every day. Well, that's a different story.

In Defense of Our Concerned Friends and Family

Before we get into how to teach our loved ones and friends how to be great supporters in our life with diabetes, let's give them a little credit first. Whether you're a kid, a high-powered attorney, or a granddaddy, the people in your life who love you and care about you have a right to be concerned about your diabetes. That's just how the world works.

Imagine for a moment that your very best friend has a serious allergy to the color blue *if* she wears more than one blue item of clothing at a time. The allergic response isn't always the same either: sometimes it just makes her seem just a little sick and other times she might seem super sick. Despite being fully aware of her allergy, at least two or three times a week she wears two or three items of blue clothing and knowingly makes herself sick. She insists it's okay, it's no big deal, because it isn't immediately life-threatening, but you still always worry about her.

Look, okay, I'll cut it out with the blue clothing allergy analogy, but please, tell me you wouldn't be concerned about friends who had an illness? Tell me you wouldn't want to watch over them, try to help them, or caution them when they were doing something you knew wasn't necessarily the best for their health and well-being?

I know there are *many* exceptions to the situation, especially when the comments come out sounding very critical, ignorant, and mean—and that's a different issue that we'll talk about later—but when you think about those around you who truly love you, truly want good things for you, and are truly worried about you and your diabetes (especially if you're struggling with your blood sugars), we need to remember that someone who loves us would never stand back and just watch us struggle and hurt ourselves.

If the tables were turned, we certainly would never stand back and watch our friends struggle and hurt themselves either, right? We'd speak up. We'd say *something*. And we may not always say the right thing, but we can't help ourselves. All we know is that our friend or girlfriend or mom or son or brother is struggling.

And lying. Oh, that's a tricky one. If we start lying to those around us about our blood sugars, then we are fueling the fire of the tense relationship and stress around diabetes management. How can the people who love us trust that we're doing our best in our diabetes management if they can't even trust that the words coming from our mouths are true? It's our responsibility to be honest.

Our friends and family *do* have a right to express their concern if they think we aren't taking good care of ourselves. They do! That's what love is, baby! Asking them to "not worry" or "say nothing" is like asking a … a bunny to stop hopping. (I know, that's silly, but just go with it). That's what friends and family do: they express concern and love, but teaching them *how* to be supportive and *how* to talk to us about our diabetes in a way that actually *feels* loving is our responsibility.

And it might not be as tricky as you think.

Five Reasons It's Challenging to Support Us as People with Diabetes

1. **Diabetes is a lot of work!** Oh man, if the people in your life read *only one thing* about diabetes, let it be this paragraph. Our blood sugars are *not* going to be perfect 100 percent of the time. An out-of-range reading, whether it be too high or too low, is simply part of our life with diabetes. So many factors and variables play into every number. The food we eat, the activity and exercise we engage in, the time of the month (for women), hormones from not getting enough sleep or going through a really stressful project at work, issues with our insulin pump, or even an expired bottle of insulin can throw our blood sugars completely out the window! So overreacting to every high or low blood sugar is not only hurtful to our feelings, it's pointless.
2. **Certain blood sugars can make us cranky.** Have you ever tried to have a real conversation with someone whose blood sugar is at 50 mg/dL or 250 mg/dL? Out-of-range blood sugars affect our brains and our energy. When we're low, our brain literally isn't getting the glucose it needs in order to function—so please put your questions or conversation on

hold until we can think straight (and hey, ask if I need a juice box while you're at it!). High blood sugars can leave us feeling like we have a bad case of the flu with fatigue and nausea. What we need most in these moments, sometimes, is a glass of water, our medications or insulin, and some private space to rest until our number comes down.

3. **You love us and want the best for us.** We get it! You would do anything in the world to make our blood sugars perfect all day—and for that, we are grateful—but right now, life with diabetes means fluctuations in blood sugars, phases of life where managing diabetes can be really hard, and we don't always want to eat the same "diabetes-friendly" foods every damn day. When you see a high blood sugar on our meters, you might want to gasp or scold us, but what we actually need is support and understanding. Period. We know you love us, but we need room to be imperfect and live life while doing the best we can with diabetes. And sometimes, our very best is less than perfect—and that needs to be okay.

4. **We're tired of being told what to do.** Instead of telling us how to eat or how often to exercise, *ask us* if we're interested in borrowing a book you have or *ask us* if we care to hear about the latest report you saw on the news about diabetes. By simply *asking permission* to share information, you're giving us control over a conversation that is focused on a very personal aspect of our lives. Chances are, we'll say, "Sure, why not, what nutrition book did you just read?" and we'll listen! By asking if we want to hear about it, you'll change the delivery of that information from a lecture or advice to simply sharing something you're interested in yourself.

5. **We already judge ourselves enough.** We already know what is or isn't considered a "good" number in the world of blood sugars, and hearing that judgment on our latest blood sugar reading from *you* only adds to the already existing guilt or stress we felt when we saw the number ourselves. It's a really personal, touchy topic for many. Asking us what our blood sugar is can feel like you just asked us for our deepest darkest secret, especially if we're struggling with our diabetes in general. Don't ask for a number, don't make a statement or judgment on the number; instead, just ask, "Is there anything I can do to support you right now?"

Like I said, loving a person with diabetes isn't easy. Let's take a closer look at what great support looks like and how to teach those around us to be awesome sources of support for our life with this darn disease.

For Ages 1 through 107 Years Old

(Any diabetic who lives longer than 107 years old gets to do what they want—no questions asked.) True support shouldn't make us feel guilty, sad, ashamed, embarrassed, or attacked—ever—even when we're doing everything wrong and ignoring all the rules and sabotaging our own health.

The funny thing about expressing love and support about diabetes is that the tiniest changes in the way a sentence is structured can make all the difference. Or simply expressing a really vague question rather than a statement or a command can completely transform how it actually feels to receive that support. Better yet: it can completely change how effective and helpful the support actually is to the person living with diabetes!

And hey, this goes both ways. In other words, as the people with diabetes, we have our own ways of being difficult to talk to about our blood sugars sometimes, right? We aren't always a total pleasure to be around!

Naturally, in our day-to-day lives, we don't need to think too carefully about the way we phrase our sentences when we're chatting with friends, and we're quick to give advice, rather than simply listen. When we hear or see a problem, we love to give advice or directions on what ought to be done to solve it. Haven't you ever heard friends talk about their frustrating relationships and told them very quickly what they ought to do before really hearing the full story or even *asking* them if they *wanted* your opinion and advice? We're all pretty guilty of this.

When it comes to diabetes, you've probably had your share of friends, family, and total strangers give you varied advice on how you ought to take care of your diabetes. Some of it actually makes sense, a lot of it is blatantly incorrect, and most of it was advice you never asked for in the first place.

Here's an example of a not-so-supportive ways to communicate around diabetes:

Diabetic Checks Blood Sugar: *"I'm at 278 mg/dL."*

Not-So-Supportive Friend: *"Oh my gosh! That's bad! How'd that happen?"*

Diabetic Checks Blood Sugar: *"I don't know. I guess I didn't get enough insulin at lunch."*

Not-So-Supportive Friend: *"Well, you shouldn't eat that again!"*

Chances are, those closest to you in your life have seen a high or low number on your meter before, right? Or if you're so afraid or tired of their responses to those numbers, maybe you've stopped checking your blood sugar in front of them to just to avoid hearing the comments.

We hear comments from those who love us about out-of-range blood sugars, not checking our blood sugar often enough, eating things that have sugar in them, drinking alcohol—oh, the list goes on and on!

In an ideal world, this is how that conversation would have gone instead:

Diabetic Checks Blood Sugar: *"I'm at 278 mg/dL."*

Not-So-Supportive Friend: *"Is there anything I can do to help?"*

Diabetic Checks Blood Sugar: *"I think I just need a glass of water (or insulin, or whatever)."*

Not-So-Supportive Friend: *"Okay. I know this is really hard work— you're doing a great job."*

But preventing those more critical comments comes down to this: taking a moment to explain to your friends and family what kind of support you actually need.

As an adult, my parents are quite removed from my daily diabetes management now. Instead, my friends and boyfriend are really the bigger supporters. At one point, early in the relationship with my boyfriend, I had to switch from taking my Lantus injection in the morning at 7:00 a.m. to taking it at night around 9:00 p.m. After *years* of taking this injection at 7:00 a.m. every day, it was very difficult for my brain to get used to the new routine! And so, I asked my boyfriend for exactly the kind of support I needed: "Hey, love, before we brush our teeth every night, would you mind asking me if I've taken my Lantus injection yet?"

And he did, for a while, until it was clear that my new routine had become "the norm" and I didn't need the daily reminder.

In some situations, though, you may have to *undo* the way someone has been expressing their concern and support for your diabetes for a long time. And that can be a tad trickier because they are so used to behaving or communicating that way about your diabetes that explaining how you'd like them to do it differently could potentially cause an argument or hurt feelings.

Instead of pointing out that they are doing something wrong, communicate the change you'd like to see by talking simply in terms of what you *need* and *want* and *feel*.

Here are a few examples, written in letter-form, that you're more than welcome to steal and use in your own life:

Dear Dan (a boyfriend),

I really appreciate how much you care about my diabetes, and I think the best way you can help me is to only offer help if I ask for it. Or if you see a number on my meter that concerns you, you can always ask, "How are you? Can I do anything for you?" Sometimes, in life with diabetes, I have highs or lows, and what I need the most is just space to wait patiently while that number comes down or goes up to a safer number. To me, that would feel like the best kind of support.

Dear Mom,

I know you love me, and you want me to check my blood sugar at least four times before I even get home from school for the day, but sometimes that pressure makes me feel very angry. I know I'm doing the best I can—and that isn't always perfect. When you react to a blood sugar on my meter with a judgment about how it's bad, I feel very criticized and embarrassed. Sometimes, what I really need to hear from you is, "Great job on taking the time to check your blood sugars. If you need any help understanding what caused the highs or lows, I'm here for you." That's what great support would feel like to me.

Dear Jenny (a friend),

I know you love me, and you want the best for me, but when you try to tell me what I can or can't eat, it feels like an invasion of my privacy. In the end, I'm responsible for what I choose to eat, and I can't eat perfectly all the time. Instead, I wish you could simply be there to listen if I do have something to share about my diabetes or nutrition. You don't need to have all the answers, I just need someone to listen. That would feel like the kind of support I really need.

Dear Mark (a brother),

I know you're concerned about my diabetes, but I need to explain that feeling pressured by you to lose weight and eat perfectly makes me feel uncomfortable. It makes me feel like I'm a failure when I'm trying really hard to make changes. Instead, the kind of support I'd really love from you is if you want to go for a walk with me every other day after work. Having you as a walking buddy would really help me exercise more often! That is the best way you could support me in my life with diabetes.

Dear Dad,

I am really struggling with my diabetes right now. I know how to take my insulin and check my blood sugar, but I wish I didn't have to do those things, and feeling constantly scolded and punished for not doing them perfectly only makes me hate my diabetes more and more and more. I need a different kind of support. I want to feel like I can turn to you when my blood sugar is high without getting scolded and blamed. Instead, I want to be able to just tell you, rather than hide it from you, and just have somebody there to say, "I know this sucks." That's the kind of support I really need right now.

Dear Elaine (a girlfriend),

You are the greatest girlfriend ever and I so appreciate that you've taken so much time to learn about my diabetes, but I think I'd like to shift a little bit in how you show your support for me. Now that I'm really in the habit of taking my insulin regularly, I think I'd rather ask you for help remembering my shot only when I feel like I might need help. In other words, you don't have to remind me anymore, I want to be responsible for remembering all on my own. If you really think I've forgotten, and you didn't see me take my shot, then I'll be grateful for the reminder. That would be the best kind of support I could ask for from you.

These letters are simple and clear and specific. They might seem painfully simple, but these are the kinds of things that genuinely need to be spelled out. Sometimes a mom or a concerned friend might be so caught up in wanting you to be as healthy as possible that they don't realize their behavior leaves you feeling like a guilt-ridden diabetic who can't do anything right! In an ideal world, we should be able to turn to those who love us and just talk about our diabetes—especially the rougher days with out-of-whack blood sugars—and feel only support, not shame or blame.

But that kind of support comes through communicating clearly. Sometimes, it's the simple difference between making accusations or making judgments about diabetes and simply asking a very sincere question: *"Is there anything I can do to help?"*

Teaching this difference to your friends and family can reduce the stress in your home and life tremendously. The next time you hear someone speaking to you about your diabetes in a way that leaves you feeling stressed, guilty, scolded, or angry, try taking a deep breath and explaining:

"Hey _____, next time, in a situation like this, what would feel more supportive to me is if you simply said, 'I know diabetes is really hard, and you're doing the best you can. Is there anything I can do to support you?'"

I know—this seems so overly simple—but it can make all the difference, and it needs to be explained clearly and calmly to the people who love you. They don't know what it's like to live with diabetes and they can't read our minds. And remember, next time you find yourself really, crazily frustrated by a friend or family's comment, remind yourself that they love you!

A Letter from Ginger to Parents of Children with Type 1 Diabetes

I don't have any children—especially any children living with type 1 diabetes. However, throughout the many years I've been chatting with, writing for, presenting to, and working with all kinds of people with all kinds of diabetes, I have developed a personal theory that I'm only more certain of after recently spending another weekend surrounded by families raising children with diabetes: raising a child with diabetes seems significantly more stressful than living with it myself.

Now I don't mean to confuse you: living with diabetes myself is not easy. It's *a lot* of work, and if it appears easy it's only because I've put so much energy into understanding the science of my body mixed with the science of diabetes over the years, and even then, my blood sugars are not perfect.

Raising a child with diabetes, rather than living with it yourself, is like asking a Mama Dog to keep a cookie balanced perfectly on top of her Puppy's nose for the rest of his youth—even while jumping around at recess—and then hope that you did a good enough job while he was a puppy that he'll grow up to be an adult dog who now knows how to balance a cookie on the top of his nose for the rest of his life.

That's a *crazy* thing to ask a Mama Dog and a Puppy to do perfectly all the time.

I can only imagine the thoughts that go through your head constantly if you're raising a young child (we'll get to teens in a moment) with diabetes:

- "How many high blood sugars does it really take for my child's future to be affected?"
- "Will she really grow up to be successful and happy like any kid without diabetes?"
- "What about our dreams for my son to be in the NBA or a professional ballerina or NASCAR driver?"
- "Is my child's life going to feel as crazy difficult as it does right now just because of this stupid disease?"
- "Will they make it through the night alive without any severe low blood sugars?"
- "Will they make good choices in college when I'm not there to look after them?"
- "Is everything going to be okay?"

I cannot imagine what it's like to be constantly worried about severe low blood sugars in a child who is too young to identify and communicate the symptoms of a low. I cannot imagine what it's like to go to sleep at night and hope and pray that everything will be okay by morning. I cannot imagine what it's like to wonder how awful your child must be feeling when you see a 357 mg/dL on his glucose meter and know it's been that high for hours.

You're the parent. You want everything to be okay, and yet, in life with diabetes, there's only so much you can do for your children.

I can tell you, as a person living with diabetes, that high and low blood sugars are not fun. Sometimes they're awful, sometimes they're not as awful, but either way, I support myself through them by *not* making them a bigger deal than they have to be.

No guilt. No blame. Or at least, as little guilt as possible.

That's where you come in. Whether your child is still relying heavily on you for all of their diabetes care or have moved into their teens and are expected to remember to check their blood sugars several times while they're at school, one of the most important aspects of preventing *their own* burnout is in how you communicate to children about their diabetes.

I can't remember how many times a parent has said to me, "John is only checking his blood sugar three times a day lately! How do I get him to check more?"

My genuine reaction to this is *not,* "Oh my gosh, only three times a day?" but instead, "Wow, your teenager is actually taking the time to think about this annoying chronic illness three times a day? That's awesome! Stop giving him a hard time and give him some credit! Give him a high-five for making a clear effort!"

Support. More support! If you raise your teen to be a person with diabetes who knows that his parents are proud of him as long as he's being honest and giving his best in any given moment (which does *not* mean perfection), then you'll raise a teen who not only doesn't resent his diabetes as much … but he won't resent his parents as much either!

Support. Support. Support.

The next time you find yourself commenting on or reacting to your child's blood sugar, ask yourself if the words that just came out of your mouth sounded supportive. I know you're concerned, you're stressed out, but the way you communicate to children or teenagers about their diabetes will absolutely impact how well they take care of themselves and how they view their life with diabetes.

Parents and kids with diabetes need to be on the same team. If you're playing *against* each other, burnout is inevitable and practically instantaneous. Being on the same team, which means no one ever scolds or blames or guilt-trips or rolls their eyes over a number, means that your child can actually turn to you for help and support rather than hide from you out of fear for being yelled at or punished when diabetes gets tough.

And better yet: there will simply be less angst.

But seriously, I want you to know that your children's future is still totally shiny and bright—especially if you raise them to be on your team and feeling proud of themselves for how they face diabetes every day, rather than ashamed or ridden with guilt.

Reacting emotionally to blood sugars, making them out to be more than just a number, will teach your child to react emotionally to those blood sugars. You are the leader. You are the example. When the team is struggling, you want to take a deep breath and stay as cool and calm as possible, teaching your child how to take some of the emotion out of diabetes, and focus instead on problem-solving and doing the best possible in any given moment.

And I want you to know that yeah, high blood sugars *suck*. Low blood sugars are *scary* and *they suck*. But life can go on. We can live a good life. We do live a good life. A great life. A real life. Our dreams can become reality. Our goals can be accomplished. We can thrive in college, do stupid things in college, date losers, fall in love, be broken-hearted, get hired, get fired, be promoted, have kids, have grandkids, run marathons, win the Olympics, win NASCAR, climb crazy-big mountains, and laugh wildly at things that are not really that funny just because we're in a really great mood, having a really great day … even in life with diabetes.

We can do anything.

Doing the best any of us can do in life with diabetes does *not* have to mean perfect blood sugars all the time. Sometimes our best is *awes*ome and sometimes it's not quite so awesome, but it's still our best in that moment. And that's okay. It has to be, because "perfection" is a crazy expectation.

I want you to know you're doing a great job, and the more you encourage your child to live his or her life with diabetes being just one of the many challenges in life to be faced, the more you're ensuring that anything is possible. Keep your chin up, give yourself and your child credit for simply facing diabetes every day.

Kids and Teens and Parents in Life with Diabetes

Raising a child—and especially a teenager—with type 1 diabetes is no easy task. That's why we've brought in the one and only Dr. Alicia McAuliffe-Fogarty.

Dr. McAuliffe-Fogarty was diagnosed with diabetes at the age of eleven, and has committed herself to improving the lives of children with diabetes. At the age of 18, in 1996, she established the Circle of Life Camp, Inc., a not-for-profit camp in Albany, NY. Currently, she is a Clinical Child Health Psychologist and serves on the Board of Directors of the Diabetes Education & Camping Association. She is the author of *Growing Up with Diabetes: What Children Want Their Parents to Know*, and is co-editor of *Camps and Mental Health: An Issue of Child and Adolescent Psychiatric Clinics*.

Here are three messages from Dr. McAuliffe Fogarty on raising children and teens with diabetes:

Remember, they are people first, not a disease

"Sometimes," Dr. McAuliffe-Fogarty explains, "I think parents have tunnel-vision. So instead of saying, 'How was soccer practice?' all they want to know is what their child's blood sugar is. Parents need to step back."

(continued)

(*continued*)

Kids and Teens and Parents in Life with Diabetes

"I'm a person first," she says. "I just happen to have diabetes. I am a person with diabetes. I am not a disease." This train of thought applies both to her feelings about using the word "diabetic" instead of "person with diabetes," and to always treating your child as though he or she is a diseased child, rather than a child who *also* lives with diabetes.

With pain medication, McAuliffe-Fogarty illustrates, you take pain medication and your pain goes away, "but with diabetes you don't see the effects of high blood sugar right away."

Punishment and nagging do *not* work

Diabetes is stressful, this we know, but when tension and stress is high, it can become easy to start bugging and nagging a person with diabetes.

"Parents need to come to a compromise," explains Dr. McAullife-Fogarty, "because constantly nagging a child to check their blood sugar is going to fuel their desire to *not* do it. Camps are great because they're no longer the outcast. Every kid there has diabetes. And of course with fluctuating hormones, teens can get depressed, have to face peer pressure and bullying—all the challenges of being a teen."

This comes back to remembering that your child or teen is in fact *a child or teen*. Whether it's over-washing the dishes or counting carbs, nagging drives people away. Period. And it leads to resentment. Become part of a team with your child instead one of their

(*continued*)

(*continued*)

Kids and Teens and Parents in Life with Diabetes

enemies by remembering that managing diabetes is a lot to ask of an adult, let alone a teenager. There needs to be some give and take, and most importantly, room for them to make mistakes without getting scolded. Encouragement and support is a much more efficient source of fuel than lectures and anger.

Ask yourself, as a parent, if you're listening to your teen

Dr. McAuliffe-Fogarty emphasizes the value of *active listening skills*. "Sometimes we don't actively listen, and we tune out because we think we know what they're going to say. Mixing diabetes and adolescence is very difficult because teenagers are walking the line of being not quite adults and not quite kids. The struggle of dependence and independence, they just want to be normal, but diabetes makes them inherently more dependent on their parents than their nondiabetic peers."

Kids, she says, are more swayed by their friends than by their parents, even when it comes to diabetes.

"You might just need a referee, and let them be the mediator. It's easy to get into the habit of punishing the teenager for diabetes-related things, but the teen doesn't want to hear what the parents have to say. Diabetes can come with a compromise, explaining to your child that "you can do whatever you want in life with diabetes, but you just have to figure out how to integrate diabetes in to your life."

We Are Lucky

In the end, we are lucky there are people in the world who love us enough to nag us … I suppose that's one perspective we could always remember. We are lucky to not be in this alone, even if those nondiabetic family and friends can't understand exactly how it feels to be lightheaded, anxious, and trembling during a low blood sugar, or nauseated and pissed off during a high. We're lucky they are in our lives at all. So, from my friends and family to yours, thank you.

What Others Have to Say: On Help

Jim Turner, living with type 1 diabetes
(YouTube.com/pillboxchannel)

For me, the most overwhelming aspect of having diabetes is low blood sugar. The big ones exhaust me and the little ones drain me. But at least with the big ones, I'll sometimes have a good story to tell after, but it's the little ones that gnaw at me, wear me down, and depress me.

There are so many moments in my life when I was low and didn't quite know what I was doing or thinking or saying—moments that are gone forever because I was not quite there. Sometimes these lows come in waves and then I really have to work to overcome the feeling that I am failing my disease and myself.

This might sound weird but I've tried to keep my wife at arm's length regarding my diabetes. She understands the basic rudiments of it, but I don't go into any detail with her—though she's scary good at recognizing when I'm going low. Sometimes I'll walk in a room, she'll just look up and say, "You need something to eat." Sometimes I argue with her, but she's usually right.

(continued)

(continued)

What Others Have to Say: On Help

And of course now that I wear a CGM, she's like an owl whenever an alarm goes off. She'll be in the other room and it'll vibrate and she'll yell, "Jim, what was that? Are you low or high?"

Brandy Barnes, living with type 1 diabetes
(DiabetesSisters.org)

My husband, Chris, is my "cushion." He always catches me when I fall—literally and figuratively—whether its from a low blood sugar, forgetting a snack, or just getting burned-out from diabetes. I think the most supportive thing he has ever done is taking over my diabetes management for an entire weekend. It was an eye-opening experience for both of us. Before you ask—yes, he had to count carbs and determine (on his own) how much insulin to dose for everything I ate. I usually get gasps from women when I say that. But it wouldn't be a true learning experience for him if I gave him all of the answers and he didn't have to do all of the "guessing" we have to do every day when it comes to carb-counting.

Also, not doing all of the calculations was a huge relief to me. Because I had never ever had someone else doing it for me, I never knew what that experience was like, to not have to use your brain for diabetes calculations! Let's just say that the calculations take up more energy than I realized. And let's just say that for a very relaxed, laid-back guy, I observed Chris becoming much more anxious during the weekend he took over my diabetes. I wasn't on a continuous glucose monitor at the time, so he was constantly checking my blood sugar. I think if you asked him, he would say that it was definitely tiring. At 5:00 p.m. (on the dot) on Sunday afternoon, he came to me and said, "Okay, the weekend is over now. I'm off duty." You could feel his sense of relief. I think it gave him a greater sense

(continued)

(continued)

What Others Have to Say: On Help

of appreciation for the work involved in diabetes and I also think it gave him a better understanding of the tightrope we walk with diabetes: counting carbs exactly right and making the right dose so that our blood sugars will stay between a particular set of numbers.

For all of the women out there: it was nice to have someone else taking care of my diabetes. It really was a break for me. However, you have to plan to do this during a time when your spouse is going to be with you the entire time—he's not planning to go play golf for four hours on Saturday afternoon or you're not planning a night out with the girls. Not always easy to plan!

Leonard Auter, living with type 2 diabetes

The most challenging aspect of life with diabetes for me is managing diabetes and work. It's not as challenging in the summer when my work hours are pretty much the same day-to-day, but during the winter, when my job changes from truck driver hauling gravel to plowing snow, my work schedule can change daily depending on the weather. Some days, I go to work at regular time and when it snows I will get the 2:00 a.m. wakeup call to get out and plow. I work late some days and some weekends, too. I do manage it pretty well with my insulin pump and continuous glucose monitor; both help manage diabetes with my type of work. I pack my breakfast and lunch so I can keep on the same eating schedule, but exercise and sleep schedule are the biggest change.

I'm pretty straightforward with my family, friends, and coworkers as a truck driver, and they are pretty well informed now about my diabetes. Every once in a while I might have to correct them. Mostly, my diabetes isn't much of an issue now. My coworkers know that I use a continuous glucose monitor, but I haven't showed them

(continued)

(continued)

What Others Have to Say: On Help

the sensor before until recently. A few weeks ago, I used my arm for a sensor site for the first time—usually it was hidden somewhere by my clothing before—and I showed it to them. They were kind of in shock at first, and I had to explain how I have to change it once a week, and yes, I do it myself, and I explained that I also have to change my pump infusion set every three days as well.

My supervisors and coworkers have been the most supportive when I'm sick, or if I have a doctor's appointment in the middle of the workday, I can call in and they won't question my need for time off. I also do my part, too, by letting them know in advance if I have an appointment coming up and by staying active and as healthy as I can so that I can pull my own weight and do my job well! If I wasn't wearing an insulin pump, no one would ever know I had diabetes based purely on my performance at work.

Cynthia Zuber, living with type 1 diabetes
(Diabeteslight.com)

I have been married five and one-half years to a loving and patient man. One of the most helpful things my husband does is that he gives me the time and space I need to take care of my health. Whether it's allowing me to go back to sleep on some mornings for a few more hours while he keeps the house quiet, washing the dishes, going to the grocery store, or cooking so that I can go on one of my long walks, attend yoga class, or rest. He has a clear understanding of the role good daily self-care plays in ensuring good health for me in the future. My health is our first priority in our marriage financially as well, and he willingly puts aside other things to pay for my medical care, organic groceries, and additional holistic treatments which help me feel my best.

(continued)

(continued)

What Others Have to Say: On Help

He also exercises with me! Not every day, but when he has time, and especially on the days I lack energy and motivation. His physical presence and support are what get me out the door sometimes. He also helps with middle-of-the-night lows by getting me orange juice if needed and setting an alarm on his iPhone if my blood sugar needs retesting. The last three years he has joined me in participating and fundraising for the ADA Tour de Cure to help find a cure for diabetes. Lastly, he provides a listening ear when needed for the times diabetes leaves me feeling fed up and at the end of my rope.

Julius Alberico, living with type 2 diabetes

As a diabetic I am married to the perfect partner. She's totally supportive and completely nonjudgmental. It's a shame that more medical professionals don't have her character. While her goal (and mine, too) would be "perfect behavior," she understands that humans aren't built that way. As a result, if I don't behave "perfectly" (yes … it happens), she doesn't make it all about her. She simply encourages me to continue trying. She's a dream to live with.

Since she supports me simply to do my best, doesn't complain, and loves me unconditionally, I am proud to say that my most recent A1C was 5.5 percent. I couldn't have done this with someone bugging me. She knows me and knows I figure things out on my own and that I hate being told what to do by *anyone*. It's all support all the time from my wonderful Pammy. She never wavers. Ever! I know I'm a lucky guy and have been for over 43 years of married life!

(continued)

(continued)

What Others Have to Say: On Help

Mike Hoskins, living with type 1 diabetes
(DiabetesMine.com)

This may sound superficial, but one of the most supportive things my wife does is carry my diabetes meter case. I have come to rely on her carrying it in her purse so much. It's actually strange to travel to conferences on my own without her, because I have to actually think about how to tote it around and not forget it. But more broadly, that's just one example of all the incredible support she offers, from reminders to diabetes-math calculations to just listening to my rants and raves about diabetes in every aspect.

Sue Rericha, living with type 2 diabetes
(Rfamhere.blogspot.com)

Once I realize I'm dealing with burnout, I try to come up with a plan. I talk to my family or some online friends for motivation. Unfortunately, sometimes I overdo the attempt of being the perfect diabetic, but I usually notice that quickly and I work at finding balance. Going for walks helps. I will also buy some of my favorite low-carb snacks. Listening to inspirational music helps me to get out of a glum mood.

My husband is a wonderfully caring man who tries to do whatever he can to help me. When I'm dealing with burnout, the best thing he does is listen. Having him listen to me as I vent my frustrations is one of the best things he can do. If he goes to the store while I'm dealing with some low moods, he'll pick up a Diet Coke just for me. It's little things that help me get through burnout. He is a great cook and makes some great low-carb meals. It's not easy balancing

(continued)

(*continued*)

What Others Have to Say: On Help

my need for low-carbs with the needs of growing children. When he catches me eating something that has a lot of carbs, he will say in a loving, teasing voice, "Bad diabetic!" I know he's not scolding. He's trying to make light of a situation that could be difficult. If my mood interprets his caring as the "diabetes police," then I'll just tell him how I feel. We've been together long enough where I can be honest with him.

Probably the hardest part of diabetes management is regulating the carbs with my activity level as the mom of five children. We're a busy group and wind up eating fast food a couple of times per week. It's hard to make those healthy choices in the drive-thru.

The easiest aspect is finding support. I do feel that support is a very important part of diabetes management. Between the diabetes online community, my husband, and my children, I have an amazing support system.

Stacey Divone, living with type 1 diabetes
(**Portablepancreasgirl.com**)

Joe is very supportive of my life with diabetes. I've had type 1 diabetes since way before I knew him so it has been part of me since the day we met. He is always making suggestions for me to overcome an obstacle whether it be diet, exercise, or blood glucose related. They may not always be suggestions that work, but he does always try, which I truly appreciate. You can tell that he wants the best for me and wants to see me do the best I can at keeping myself healthy. Luckily, he is fitness-oriented so that has helped a lot over the years in overcoming my exercise struggles.

(*continued*)

(*continued*)

What Others Have to Say: On Help

According to him, he doesn't necessarily feel burned-out when it comes to my diabetes (although I'm certain there must be times when he does!), but instead, frustrated. Frustrated that he can't really do anything for me or seeing the frustration that I sometimes go through. But he knows it is part of the deal and copes with it the best way he knows how.

Ryan Kellan, living with type 2 diabetes

At first, my diagnosis was incredibly stressful for my wife. She does most of the cooking so she felt like she had to take on all the responsibility of learning about all these food changes. To help lighten the load, so to speak, we started learning about the nutrition together and even, for a while, we did the grocery shopping together so it wasn't all on her to plan meals for the week.

The most helpful thing she does, aside from all the food prep, is bringing my meter and insulin to my chair where I'm always sitting before dinner. She always brings it to me and so for that one part of the day, I don't have to remember. It may seem like a small thing, but it means a lot in the end.

But she does worry. When my numbers are running higher because I've been eating more sweets, or when we had to up my medication doses, she worried. I am not a perfect diabetic and I definitely don't follow all the rules, and that stresses her out. You can't blame her, she wants me to live a long time! I know not to take her worry as criticism, and instead remind myself that she just loves me, and wants to grow old with me. That's okay. I can't complain about being loved and wanted!

What Others Have to Say: On Having Children with Diabetes

Melissa Elstad, mom of Jon, diagnosed with type 1 diabetes at age two

For myself, when I am feeling burned-out it is usually because I feel I am doing everything right: counting carbs, picking foods that are healthy and have the least erroneous impact on Jon's sugars, keeping ahead of supply orders and doctor appointments—but then we still have crazy unexpected highs or lows that make me feel like a failure and fear for my sons future health. I become depressed, self-critical, and scared. I try not to show these emotions to Jon as I do not want him to feel that way when he is older and more independent with his care.

For my husband, he gets angry. He wonders "Why our Jonny?"

How do we deal with it as parents? We express our feelings to each other as appropriate (without upsetting Jon). We accept that there is no alternative. We do our best to manage it because otherwise its complications will creep up and start to manage him. We remind ourselves that allowing that blood sugar reading to dictate our happiness will become exhausting—since he is currently tested approximately 15 times a day due to complete hypoglycemia and hyperglycemia unawareness. We accept the number for what it is and do our best to get it back to where it should be ... hoping to figure why it happened is great, but rarely possible.

For Jon, he shows some anger, some sadness, some exhaustion. He has said things like: "When are the scientists going to find a cure for me?" "Why doesn't my brother have this, too?" "I am sick of this and don't want it anymore!" "If we change my name will it go away?" "I'm sick of testing myself—I do it all the time." "I'm done with this—no more site changes, it hurts." "Please make it go away."

(continued)

(continued)

What Others Have to Say: On Having Children with Diabetes

We listen and share that we feel the same way for him. We never discount his feelings or tell him to "get over it." We explain that as frustrating as it is we have to stay strong and not let diabetes win! At age six, he of course enjoys when we talk about how he is so brave and strong like a superhero! We speak positively about the scientists and how they are getting so close to a cure. We do not usually "limit" him, or treat him differently than his brother. If we are at a birthday party, Jon doesn't sit and have a sugar-free popsicle while everyone else has cake (which is something we did do per our first endocrinologist's recommendation). To see his reaction to that as a two-year-old was heartbreaking. As parents we believe that if we restrict him all the time, he will retaliate when he's older. We want him to be just like a lot of people: to make many healthy choices, but to "live a little," too.

John Franklin, father of Cade, diagnosed with type 1 diabetes at age four

There are so many factors that come into play as your child grows and matures. A lot of outside influences due to school, peers, sports, etc. Also, as they mature, there is a balancing act of independence versus taking over. You need to listen to them at times. When our son says that he feels better playing soccer at a lower blood sugar level than he did previously, we make a note and change accordingly. On the flip side, they are kids, and they aren't aware of the consequences of their choices yet. The judgment call has to be able to balance what is ultimately good for their well-being, while not being overbearing and making it into a life-long chore that they will resent.

Every waking moment you worry. It's not just providing food, clothing and shelter … it's literally keeping them alive. It's your Watch. Your Job. Your Child.

(continued)

(*continued*)

What Others Have to Say: On Having Children with Diabetes

If you take that into consideration, you literally become a sympathetic diabetic. You feel what they feel. You *want* to take that feeling of a high or low away. Your mind and actions are on AutoPilot, you do what needs to be done, whenever it needs to be done. You don't think twice, you don't hesitate. They need it; you supply it.

Now, that level of alertness takes its toll without any regard to your personal health. There is a theory that states that you need to take care of yourself first, before you take care of others. That is pure fiction because we would (and do) gladly sacrifice our own well-being for our children.

Your lack of sleep, weight fluctuations, the overwhelming sense of simply not knowing or second-guessing yourself and your spouse about the choices that are made can wreak havoc on any and all aspects of marriage, parenthood, and self-esteem.

As a guy, my normal inclination is to fix things. As a parent of a child with diabetes, that feeling is multiplied exponentially. You can't fix this. I'll say it again: you can't fix this. Now, try to tell yourself that after everything that you have been taught, shown, believe, and hold dear. Better yet, try to admit defeat to yourself when you look at your child while not letting them know. You can't. So you hop back on the roller coaster/treadmill that is your life and try to stop it … or at least slow it down a bit … two minutes … five minutes … nope not going to happen. All the time your mind is racing, trying to find a clue to a riddle that has no answer. And this happens … all day … every day.

That is what burnout is to me. Mental exhaustion, physical pain, and a keen sense of not being able to make it better.

(*continued*)

(continued)

What Others Have to Say: On Having Children with Diabetes

My advice? Don't hate diabetes. Respect the hell out of it. Don't waste valuable energy hating something that you cannot change … or fix. And please do not show your frustration in front of your children. They are a lot more in tune with the vibe than we give them credit for being. They know. I cannot put that level of guilt on their shoulders, especially since they aren't responsible for having it. Try your best, as that's all you can do.

And breathe.

Meri Schuhmacher, mother of Jack, Ben, and Luke, diagnosed with type 1 diabetes at ages eight months, five years old, and two years old

(Ourdiabeticlife.com)

As a parent, when my child is okay, I am okay. When I see diabetes start to affect my child, that's when the hurt finds its way to the surface. Guilt is also a big factor. I am responsible for the well-being of my children. If their numbers are off, than that is on me. It is easily argued that diabetes is responsible for off numbers, but when you are knee deep in insulin adjustments its hard not to take those numbers personally. One day my children will grow up and I want to look into their eyes and say, "I did my best." A future with complications is my biggest fear.

Back in the day, I was drowning as I tried to tackle diabetes all by myself. As soon as I reached out to family and friends to help me, my load instantly lightened. It isn't easy to ask for help, but when you do, everything changes. I also find support through blogging and other online communities. It is quite freeing to lay all your

(continued)

(continued)

What Others Have to Say: On Having Children with Diabetes

frustrations out there for others to see, and then to have them comment back to you in echoes of support and validation. I call it, "the power of same." Knowing we aren't alone, and knowing that others are running the same marathon makes all the difference. There is nothing more crushing than feeling alone and unsupported in all you do.

My children like to forget they have diabetes when they are overwhelmed. It isn't often they complain about diabetes … I suppose having multiple brothers with type 1 doesn't lend itself to the woe-is-me mentality. So instead they "forget." They forget to check their blood sugars. They forget to bolus before they eat. They forget to do a set change until their reservoir is empty. Apathy is our number one form of frustration and a sure sign of burnout in our household. I only just realized the connection of apathy and burnout. I would wonder how children who've had diabetes almost their entire lives would forget to bolus for breakfast. Now I understand it is a sign of struggle, not laziness. (Well, *sometimes* laziness … they are boys after all.)

I will often echo back to them their feelings. "I am tired of diabetes, too. I wouldn't want another set change either." I try to make them feel understood more than anything. And if I don't understand mentally, I try to emotionally see the battle they fight every day.

I try to treat diabetes like any other chore. It is something that needs to be taken care of, and that is non-negotiable. I'll often talk about consequences in everything that we do. Every one of our actions yields positive or negative consequences, diabetes is no different. There have been times when I let the guilt of what my

(continued)

What Others Have to Say: On Having Children with Diabetes

children go through cloud my judgment. But bad day or not, set changes need to happen. Blood sugars need to be checked. Insulin needs to be dispensed. When I see my boys in serious burnout I lend a hand as much as I can. I'll check their sugars before they wake up so that doesn't have to be the first thing they do in the morning. I'll grab their pump as they sit down to breakfast and bolus for them, or I'll call, or text them to remind them to bolus. Another thing that helps is letting them voice their frustrations. I let them tell me that "diabetes is stupid," and I'll agree with them wholeheartedly. Keeping all of this in context and at the same time not making diabetes a bigger deal than it needs to be is a delicate job for sure. All I can do is love them my best and try my best. The rest will work itself out in the wash.

Diane Pridmore, mom to Andrew (aka Batman) diagnosed with type 1 diabetes at age three
(BlueHeelSociety.org)

When my son was diagnosed with diabetes, I had just given birth to my fourth child, who was five weeks old. It was chaos learning to count carbohydrates, do a sliding scale, dilute insulin, give shots correctly, and learn what hypoglycemia looked like. Absolute chaos. I have four kids. One in a car with his newly minted license, one with diabetes, one on potty training in a preschool with no nurse, and a new baby. I don't think I slept more than a couple of hours a night for about six months. When we pushed to get him on the insulin pump, I honestly believed that *this* would get better. I believed that with our endocrinologist team, and my desire to make his life, and our lives, more "normal," it would get better. I spent countless hours

(*continued*)

(continued)

What Others Have to Say: On Having Children with Diabetes

reading, reaching out to other parents who lived this life, and challenged myself to make it my mission to not only survive mentally, but to accomplish something I could be proud of, and that was to see my son *thrive* despite his diagnosis.

We are now three years and a couple of months out from diagnosis, and while I never could foresee what lay ahead, it simply got better. It is easier, but it isn't easy. I don't want to paint a picture that managing a disease in another person, a child, my child, that has some rather barbaric devices, or that has no rules, is easy. It's very challenging. But, our day-to-day is easier. We, as a family, accept this disease as part of our normal, and my son doesn't allow it to affect him aside from the annoying interruptions for fingersticks or treatment of a low blood glucose. I learn every day from him how to just "put it on a lily pad, and let it float down the river." I don't know how it happened, but one day, I forgot about the pain and despair of his diagnosis, and just enjoyed watching him be an amazing, now, seven year old. I wish I knew then, what I know now. It gets better.

That being said … burnout? I have it. Often. As a parent, my job is to clip fingernails, make sure everyone is eating their fruits and veggies, and teaching silly songs. Hugs, kissing boo boos, finding lost toys, not swearing out loud when I step on a Lego … I wear many hats. I never intended to practice medicine on my son. The toils of changing sites, or finding correct basal rates, and just knowing the terminology, teaching it to others, writing 504 plans to keep him safe at school, teaching his baseball coach what "low" looks like, and explaining to him that being teary at 2:00 a.m., and not knowing why, or that at age seven, wetting his bed because of a high blood sugar is okay, and not his fault … it's exhausting. And most days, I want

(continued)

(*continued*)

What Others Have to Say: On Having Children with Diabetes

off the ride. But I catch glimpses of him, tubing all hanging out of his pump belt, no shirt on, riding his bike, *free* of any worry. So what the hell is *my* problem?

But I needed to talk about diabetes. He can say whatever he wants about his disease, and he has carte blanche to do so, but I do not ever talk about my feelings with him. *That* is why I needed an outlet. I needed to do diabetes my way. I helped to create an online little advocacy campaign to talk about diabetes, proper, and to have a safe place to be me, the good, the bad, and the ugly. And the Blue Heel Society was born.

It saved my life. I met thousands of parents and people who live with or care for and love someone with diabetes, and I found my family. Suddenly, I had a voice, and they all spoke my language. Homecoming, my friend. I was home. My kids will thank me one day for being crazy online and keeping it out of our living room.

I Did Everything I'm Supposed to Do and I'm Still Not Perfect

8

Embracing Your Progress and Giving Yourself Credit for Dealing with Diabetes Every Day

The funny thing about diabetes (actually, it's not that funny) is that even when we're doing everything we're supposed to do, our blood sugars aren't necessarily perfect. Literally, a few hours before the moment I wrote this very sentence, I had a snack of red grapes and pecans—a rather healthy snack, I'm sure most dietitians would agree—but an hour later my blood sugar was at 230 mg/dL because grapes, as I've mentioned earlier, just wreak havoc on my blood sugar if I don't manage to consume the mysteriously perfect amount of grapes with the mysteriously perfect amount of insulin.

And that was annoying, sure, but I think what makes me feel the most *tired* in life with diabetes is all the thinking. When I actually stop for a moment and notice just how much time I spend *thinking* about my diabetes, I feel overwhelmed. Angry. And tired.

Thinking. Worrying. Wondering. Hoping. Planning. Preparing. Calculating. Guessing. Fixing. Reacting. Fixing again. Worrying. Worrying. Worrying.

Giving most of our effort to our diabetes management *doesn't* guarantee that our blood sugars will be *mostly* perfect most of the time—there are simply too many other variables happening. Some we can control with a lot of hard work and some we cannot. Either way, the whole ordeal gets tiring day after day after day because diabetes never goes away.

It's always there. Even on the great days, even on the I-can-stand-this day, diabetes is *always* there. And I really wish it wasn't. Sometimes, even on those "perfect" days where my blood sugar actually does what I want it to, I just want to scream, "Diabetes is so stupid! So lame! So dumb! I hate it! Go away! GO. AWAY."

Nothing in particular really sparks this, it's just always there, somewhere in the background of my brain, and every now and then, it creeps more to the front, and it takes just a moment. I mean, sure, certain things could set it off—sometimes it's something small and silly like when a random person I hardly know decides to inform me that I can cure my diabetes by eating more exotic hemp seed oil from the Amazon jungle combined with regular exercise. Those kinds of comments are annoying and usually laughable, but when they're accidentally piled on top of an already challenging day of diabetes management, they might push you to the point of being truly angry.

Other days, it could be triggered by simply scheduling a routine appointment with the eye doctor where you're reminded again that every day of your life *today* will determine whether you still have your vision, fingers, toes, and kidneys down the road. That every second, every minute, every hour has an impact, good or bad, on your life because of your blood sugar level.

That is tiring. I'm tired from just typing it.

Sometimes, I get an overwhelming feeling of disgust toward diabetes for just being there. For simply existing in my life. Because it's so much work—every day. Just like I wish people didn't have to deal with cancer, leukemia, Crohn's disease, depression, hemophilia, cystic fibrosis, hearing impairments, blindness, or Down syndrome, I wish none of us had to deal with diabetes every day. But that long list of other diseases reminds me that I'm definitely not alone in my daily challenge of living with a chronic illness.

And then, somewhere in another part of my brain, a little voice says, "Okay, that's fine. You can hate your diabetes today. You can call it names. Swear at it. Resent it. Loathe and despise it. You can even get a little sloppy with your insulin doses or your carbohydrate-counting if you need to, for a moment. And then, *Ginger, darling*, you've gotta deal with it, because it isn't going away, and your life is important."

I'm not saying that's the voice *you* are supposed to hear, but that's what happens in my brain on a regular basis. A voice that is much louder than my frustration for my diabetes speaks up and reminds me that my desire to live will always outweigh my anger toward my diabetes.

The Ebb and Flow of Life with Diabetes

Take diabetes out of your head for a moment, and simply think about the rest of your life so far. Have you spent the past five, six, seven years in only one "phase" of being really happy or really challenged by everything else in your life? Probably not. Instead, you've probably had months or a couple of years where everything felt like it was going very smoothly, and then you've probably had a few months or a year where everything felt really hard.

Perhaps I simply haven't met them yet, but so far I don't know of anyone in the world whose life is always on the positive upswing! I don't know anyone who has spent the past five years in a happy glow from everything being perfect and easy. (If you think you know someone who is always living a wonderful life, I'd challenge that thought by suggesting you don't actually know them well enough. Everyone faces challenges!)

Life has an ebb and flow to it, and so does diabetes.

Sure, there are people who have put a great deal into their diabetes management so the ebbs and flows don't look all that different from each other, but even the most on-their-game diabetics I know go through phases.

What's the secret? Being okay with the ebb and flow and embracing the fact that no one's life rides perfectly on a positive note throughout their entire life. We all have ups and downs.

I believe strongly that the way we manage and perceive our own life with diabetes is simply the same as the way we approach any other things or events in our life. Some people, with or without diabetes, are enthusiastic and happy and pick themselves up quickly when life gets hard. Some people don't. Some people feel defeated easily by little or big challenges they encounter in life, and some people are born with or develop a level of resiliency that helps them keep their chin up when life gets hard. We essentially choose to be one or the other through the attitude and perspective with which we view our own life and everything that happens to us. Diabetes is simply part of that mix.

If you are a parent, which type of person are you? Are you the person who views a challenge as an obstacle that you'll work hard to climb over, or a roadblock that stops you completely? How is your child learning to face challenges through your example?

In the end, how you face diabetes will come down to a conscious decision. Have a short conversation with some of the most successful people living with diabetes, and all of them will tell you that they consciously choose to think positively about their life with diabetes. They consciously choose to see diabetes as an obstacle they will climb over with arduous effort and hard work, even enjoying the challenge, rather than resenting the challenge or seeing it as a roadblock. We can *choose* to take on diabetes.

Now you might be thinking, "*Puhleeeeeze, don't tell me I need to just 'change my mind' in order to get over my burnout.*"

Fear not: that's not what I'm saying.

You can still be burned-out while making a conscious effort to think positively about the obstacle in your life known as "diabetes." You can even choose to think positively about the ebb and flow of your burnout.

Look at the difference—or rather, *feel* the difference—of these two thoughts:

1. I'm so burned-out! Diabetes sucks. I'm so bad at diabetes.
2. I'm so burned-out. I'm doing the best I can … this is a rough week for me, just gotta work through it.

You can feel burned-out and embrace the fact that life ebbs and flows, and diabetes is part of that ebb and flow. It's okay. It's okay to have a rough week, a horrible day, a lousy month. It's okay.

And sometimes, part of embracing the ebb and flow means knowing when it's time for a diabetes vacation!

It's Time for a Diabetes Vacation!

Now, don't get your hopes up, I am not about to announce a new technique for getting your blood sugars to manage themselves while you lie on the beach for a week in Hawaii. Instead, I'm talking about planning to back off from your diabetes care in a way that is safe and thoughtful.

Just as we talked about *anticipating* burnout rather than getting frustrated with ourselves for experiencing it, we can also *plan* a diabetes vacation that might simply last a few hours, a full day, or even a few days.

A diabetes vacation gives you the freedom to be far less than perfect, even aiming for far less than perfect, while not putting your life in any immediate danger.

For example, during the week when my fella and I were packing up our condo and waiting for a closing date (that came at the very last second) on the house we were anxiously hoping to move into, my blood sugars were less than stellar. My priorities were totally elsewhere and the mental energy I had left for diabetes was limited.

But I expected this. I told myself it was okay. I even told myself, "Okay, I know this is gonna be a stressful week, so I'm gonna give myself a treat by backing off on my usual blood sugar goals."

And I planned to take a break from overly attentive diabetes care by using that week as a diabetes vacation week. I didn't cook as much fresh food, we ate gluten-free pizzas and Chinese take-out, I did my best to check my blood sugar often and take the right amount of insulin, but I didn't beat myself up for running around 200 to 250 mg/dL during several afternoons or evenings.

Of course, my vacation came at a time when other stressful things were happening, but *your vacation* might come at a time when other aspects of your life are relaxed and calm. Not because other aspects of life are stressful, but because you simply need a break from the daily mental grind of diabetes management.

What a diabetes vacation *is NOT*:

- It does not risk your immediate health or threaten to land you in the hospital.
- It does not involve skipping your insulin or oral medication doses.
- It does not involve bingeing uncontrollably on food that could raise your blood sugars to dangerously high levels.

You see, a diabetes vacation has a "Start date" and an "End date." It has a planned length of time, and a clear plan of how exactly you're going to back-off from diabetes management.

A diabetes vacation is created as a way to take a brief mental breather from the daily demands of diabetes without throwing diabetes management entirely out the window.

A diabetes vacation is a realistic, planned, thoughtful, safe way to back-off a bit from diabetes management because nobody in life with diabetes does it perfectly all the time and most of us need a sort of "break" from the daily pursuit of perfection.

What a diabetes vacation can look like:

- Enjoying more carbohydrate-based foods that you otherwise avoid, with your insulin, but without the pressure or guilt if your blood sugar is a little high afterwards.
- Checking your blood sugar less often during the day for a day or two.
- Asking a loved-one to be in charge of checking your blood sugar every night before bed.
- Eating a few of the foods you usually avoid because they can temporarily raise your blood sugars more than healthier foods, while still ensuring that you take your medications.
- Doing everything you usually do in diabetes management *without* the extra stress of expecting perfection or in-range blood sugars.

In a nutshell, a diabetes vacation is a responsible way of backing off on whatever pressure you usually put upon yourself about diabetes management. For some, it's about exercise or food, for others it's about seeing the right numbers on their glucose meter. Whatever kind of pressure you put on yourself, think about how you could back off for a day or an entire weekend—as long as it doesn't impose any immediately dangerous health risks.

Less Criticism, More Credit

Chances are, I've never even met you, but I bet you're doing a better job in life with diabetes than you're giving yourself credit for.

The following is an example of a conversation I have had with handfuls of my diabetes coaching clients:

> *Ginger: So how did the past week go?*
>
> *Person Living with Diabetes: Ehh, not so great.*
>
> *Ginger: Tell me about it.*
>
> *Person Living with Diabetes: Well, I didn't go to the gym as many times as I said I would and I ate pizza and a bunch of other junk last Sunday.*
>
> *Ginger: Okay ... what else happened?*
>
> *Person Living with Diabetes: Well, when I did go to the gym, I did my new workout from start to finish and it was great. I felt really good. And throughout the week I made really great choices about food, stuck to my carbohydrate totals for the day, and my blood sugars were pretty awesome.*
>
> *Ginger: Okay ... so for most of the week you accomplished your goals, and on Sunday you had a cheat day?*
>
> *Person Living with Diabetes: Yeah ...*
>
> *Ginger: Sounds like a pretty successful week to me!*

We are so quick to criticize ourselves and only see the things we didn't do rather than our many great choices and many great accomplishments! The result? We think we're failing and thus we lose our drive to keep going and our motivation simply because we're convinced we aren't making any progress! But progress doesn't have to happen *all the time* in 100 percent of what we do! Progress is about small steps, small moments, and small choices that lead to the big results over time.

Whether you live with diabetes yourself or you are a person who supports someone else living with diabetes, take a look at how often you criticize yourself rather than give yourself credit for everything you face every day.

A few facts about people with diabetes that deserve more credit:

1. You are working to balance something 24 hours a day that is nearly impossible to balance.
2. Even if you check your blood sugar and see a high number, you get credit for actually taking the time to prick your finger and put blood on that strip in a world that isn't exactly designed to support the needs of diabetes.
3. Even if you find yourself high after eating something considered "high-carb" or not-so-diabetes-friendly, you deserve credit for checking your blood sugar. You do!
4. You deserve credit for waking up every day and being responsible for the many things in life everyone is responsible for *while* working so hard to achieve in-range blood sugars.
5. When you're low at work or with your kids or at the gym, you deserve credit for having to function and operate and *live* while enduring a low blood sugar.
6. When you're high at work or with your kids or at the gym, you deserve credit for having to function and operate and *live* while enduring a high blood sugar.
7. You deserve credit for the zillions of times you've pricked your fingers, launched an infusion site into your flesh, or given yourself another injection.
8. You deserve credit for remembering to take your various medications.
9. Whether you checked your blood sugar two times or six times, you deserve credit for checking at all. You do!
10. You deserve credit for simply showing up. Diabetes is hard work. Every day. And you showed up.

And sure, at some point we need to look honestly at what we're doing and where we want to improve, but we all tend to focus on that part. What we don't do enough is acknowledge what we *already* do, what we're doing really well, and where we're making progress even with the smallest steps.

Take a moment to write down 10 things you've done lately or continue to do really well for yourself in your life with diabetes:

_____

_____

_____

_____

_____

_____

_____

_____

_____

_____

Fuel your own source of motivation by giving yourself less criticism and way more credit.

I Seriously Wish *YOU* and I Didn't Have Diabetes

Even with the many amazing relationships and rewarding experiences that diabetes has brought into my life, I really wish I didn't have diabetes. For all I know, I would've never joined a gym where I eventually set records as a powerlifter, or met my fella Roger and my three closest friends if I didn't have diabetes.

I wish I didn't have to count carbohydrates. Inject my flesh a bajillion times a day and prick my poor worn-out fingers a million-zillion times a day. I wish I could just head out the door with my dogs without worry about my blood sugar, or go to sleep at night without having to stop and ensure that I won't die in my sleep from a low blood sugar.

I wish that the thought of "I want to have a baby" didn't have to be accompanied by "Oh my gosh, I have to make sure my diabetes is *perfect* before I do that" and worry about ten hundred other things that I wouldn't have to worry about before, during, and after pregnancy if I didn't have diabetes.

I wish I didn't have to spend so much time thinking about my future health. My eyes. My fingers. My toes. My kidneys. My liver. My everything.

I wish *you* didn't have diabetes.

But here we are. Totally diabetic. Totally people with diabetes.

The way I see it, there are some things in life we can make a big fuss about and actually change. For instance, I am *horrible at math*. Throughout elementary school I was always in the bottom of the food-chain when it came to math classes, usually coming home with Cs and Ds on my report card but with an A+ on everything else. So what did I do when I was required to take a terrifying challenging (for me) math class that made absolutely no sense to my brain in college? I got out of it—a class that all of my peers had to take, I found a way out. I changed my circumstances. I put on my very best performance for the Director of the Professional Writing program (my major) and my academic counselor, and convinced them that the math class was a complete waste of my time.

But I can't do that with diabetes. I can't talk my way out of it. I can't ignore it. I can't pretend it's not there. I can't hide from it or run away. Trying to do any of *those* things is actually just a waste of my time, because my diabetes is not going to go away. The more I allow myself to get angry about my diabetes, the more energy I'm simply wasting on being angry. What good will it do me to invest loads of my energy resenting something that I can't change? In fact, the more I pay attention to it, the less intrusive it becomes. The less it interferes with my goals and dreams. The less it gets in the way of life.

Fighting the reality of my diabetes would be like fighting the reality of the freckles all over my nose.

I wish it wasn't so. For you and for me. But here we are, with diabetes as real as freckles.

Every morning (and sometimes in the middle of the night or the crack of dawn), we wake up to face diabetes again. It's another day of pills, injections, and blood sugars. Another day of counting carbs or avoiding carbs or feeling guilty over carbs or tediously trying to balance all the carbs. Another day of tiring highs or trembling, sweaty lows. Another day of raised eyebrows and rude comments and endless questions (and hopefully some awesome support sometimes, too!). Another day. And then, we wake up and get to face it all again.

In some ways, the whole "wake up and face it all again" is obviously an exhaustingly stressful reality, but in other ways, it's kind of like shaking an Etch-a-Sketch. Whatever happened yesterday doesn't matter. Today is a new day.

It's a fact: diabetes is part of my life, and your life, whether we like it or not, right? When we wake up, it's there. I believe embracing that fact makes it easier. Working with it, rather than against it, makes it easier. Acknowledging that it's hard and giving myself credit on a daily basis, rather than resenting the demands of diabetes, helps fuel the confidence I have in my ability to face diabetes every day.

I wish we didn't have diabetes. I really do. I also wish and hope and believe that we're able to face it, deal with it, and even find inspiration in it. This disease we never asked for. Take a deep breath and simply do the best we can do.

It's okay to be tired. Burned-out. Exhausted. Even angry. It really is okay. But we can't stop or give up. Every day, we've gotta show up and do the best we can do.

Resources

Contributors

- Andy Holder, eight-time Ironman Triathlon finisher, living with type 1 diabetes. InsulinNation.com
- Allison Nimlos, living with type 1 diabetes. TheBloodSugarWhisperer.wordpress.com
- Asha Brown, living with type 1 diabetes. WeAreDiabetes.org
- Beatriz Dominguez, living with type 2 diabetes. CrankyPancreas.com
- Bethany Rose, living with type 1 diabetes. MewithD.wordpress.com
- Bradford Gildon, amateur elite triathlete, living with type 1 diabetes. TuDiabetes.org
- Brandy Barnes, living with type 1 diabetes. DiabetesSisters.org
- Brian Cohen, living with type 2 diabetes. TuDiabetes.org/profile/bsc
- Bob Pederson, living with type 2 diabetes. Tminustwo.net
- Catherine Vancak, professional dancer, living with type 1 diabetes. DanceThruBeetus.blogspot.com
- Cynthia Zuber, living with type 1 diabetes. DiabetesLight.com
- Diane Pridmore, mom to Andrew, diagnosed with type 1 diabetes at age three. BlueHeelSociety.org
- Gary Scheiner, Certified Diabetes Educator, living with type 1 diabetes. IntegratedDiabetes.com
- Jill Meisen, marathon runner, living with type 2 diabetes. Hudsuckerproxy.blogspot.com
- Jim Onwiler, avid cyclist, living with type 1 diabetes.
- Jim Turner, living with type 1 diabetes. YouTube.com/pillboxchannel
- John Franklin, father of Cade, diagnosed with type 1 diabetes at age four.
- Julius Alberico, living with type 2 diabetes.
- Kate Cornell, living with type 2 diabetes. Kates-Sweet-Success.blogspot.com
- Leonard Auter, living with type 2 diabetes.
- Melissa Elstad, mom of Jon, diagnosed with type 1 diabetes at age two.
- Meri Schuhmacher, mother of Jack, Ben, and Luke, diagnosed with type 1 diabetes at ages eight months, five years old, and two years old. Ourdiabeticlife.com

- Mike Durbin, living with type 2 diabetes and congestive heart failure. MyDiabeticHeart.com
- Mike Hoskins, living with type 1 diabetes. DiabetesMine.com
- Phyllisa Deroze, living with type 2 diabetes. DiagnosedNotDefeated.com
- Riva Greenberg, living with type 1 diabetes. DiabetesStories.com
- Ryan Attar, CrossFit coach, living with type 1 diabetes. 1HappyDiabetic.com
- Scott Strange, living with type 1 diabetes. StrangelyDiabetic.com
- Stacey Divone, living with type 1 diabetes. Portablepancreasgirl.com
- Sue Rericha, living with type 2 diabetes. Rfamhere.blogspot.com
- Terena Wilkens, avid cyclist, living with type 2 diabetes.
- Ward Alper, living with type 2 diabetes. TheDecadentDiabetic.com
- Will Dubois, diabetes educator, living with type 1 diabetes. LifeAfterDX.Blogspot.com

Mental Health Contributors

- **Dr. Alicia McAuliffe-Fogarty, living with type 1 diabetes. CircleofLifeCamp.org**
  Dr. McAuliffe-Fogarty was diagnosed with diabetes at the age of 11, and has committed herself to improving the lives of children with diabetes. At the age of 18, she established the Circle of Life Camp, Inc., a not-for-profit camp in Albany, NY, in 1996. Currently, she is a clinical child health psychologist and serves on the Board of Directors of the Diabetes Education & Camping Association. She completed her Fellowship at the Yale Child Study Center/ Yale University School of Medicine. She is the author of *Growing Up with Diabetes: What Children Want Their Parents to Know*, co-editor of *Camps and Mental Health: An Issue of Child and Adolescent Psychiatric Clinics*, and has published many articles. Dr. McAuliffe-Fogarty has received several awards for her efforts to improve the lives of children with diabetes. She currently resides in Westchester, NY, with her husband and daughter.

- **Dr. Jen Nash, living with type 1 diabetes. PositiveDiabetes.com**
  Dr. Nash is a clinical psychologist, chartered with the British Psychological Society, living with type 1 diabetes since childhood. Motivated to provide emotional support to individuals struggling with the condition, in 2009 she founded Positive Diabetes, a therapy and education service to address the psychological impact of living with type 1 and type 2 diabetes, and recently published the book *Diabetes and Wellbeing*. Nash offers support

worldwide, via Skype. To find out more and obtain a free self-help book, visit her website.

- **Leann Harris, certified positive psychology coach, living with type 1 diabetes. DelphiDiabetesCoaching.com**
Leann Harris has lived with type 1 diabetes and autoimmune disorders since 2000. She works as a diabetes coach at DelphiDiabetesCoaching .com using positive psychology and cognitive behavior techniques to address the emotional and social aspects of living with diabetes, such as anxiety, fear, relationship, and life challenges. Her passion is to help others by starting where they are now to creatively move forward, and maximize each person's strengths to uncover possibilities. Her decade of experience as a health care analyst has also helped her to understand the complexities of the government and insurance industry on health, and works to empower people to become their own medical advocates. As an educator, she works to share resources and improve life for all types of diabetics.

Websites

- DiabetesDaily.com
- TuDiabetes.org
- ParentingDiabeticKids.com
- ChildrenwithDiabetes.com
- DiabetesAdvocates.org
- DiabetesCAF.org
- YouCanDoThisProject.com
- MyGlu.org
- BehaviorialDiabetesInstitute.org
- IntegratedDiabetes.com
- DiabulimiaHelpline.com

Books

- Alicia McAuliffe-Fogarty. 1998. *Growing Up with Diabetes.* Hoboken, NJ: Wiley.
- Gary Scheiner. 2012. *Think Like a Pancreas.* New York: Da Capo Lifelong Books.

- Ginger Vieira. 2011. *Your Diabetes Science Experiment*. Fairfax, VA: Living in Progress Publishing.
- Ginger Vieira. 2012. *Emotional Eating with Diabetes*. Fairfax, VA: Living in Progress Publishing.
- Jen Nash. 2013. *Diabetes and Wellbeing*. Hoboken, NJ: Wiley-Blackwell.
- Leighann Calentine. 2012. *Kids First, Diabetes Second*. Ann Arbor, MI: Spry Publishing.
- Mark Hyman. 2008. *The Ultra-Mind Solution*. New York: Scribner.
- Mark Hyman. 2012. *Blood Sugar Solution*. New York: Little, Brown & Company.
- Michael Pollan. 2009. *In Defense of Food*. New York: Penguin Books.
- Moira McCarthy. 2013. *Raising Teens with Diabetes*. Ann Arbor, MI: Spry Publishing.
- William Polonsky. 1999. *Diabetes Burnout*. Alexandria, VA: American Diabetes Association.

Index